Revitalized

A new rendering of Charlotte Mason's *School Education*

by

Anne E. White

Cover design and photo by Bryan White

ISBN: 978-1-990258-12-1

Table of Contents

Dedication

For Wendi, because it always was for her.

Before the Curtain Rises

When I was six years old, I was taken to Toronto to see the National Ballet perform Tchaikovsky's *Sleeping Beauty*.

For those unfamiliar with this ballet, it was first staged in 1890, with choreography by Marius Petipa. It's Tchaikovsky's longest ballet: performed in full with intermissions, the performance can take up to four hours. The 1972 staging was specially adapted by Rudolf Nureyev, who added some new choreography (especially for his own part of Prince Florimund). It was gorgeously produced, full of lavish costumes and sets.

And what did a small, near-sighted six-year-old sitting far back in the theater make of all that spectacle?

To be honest, I almost fell asleep during the Prologue. The stage was crowded with brightly-robed members of the royal court (plus the fairies and so on), but I thought it was very long and boring. What I wanted to see most was the Famous Ballerina, Veronica Tennant, who didn't come on stage until Act I. And what I remembered best afterward was the Bluebird *pas de deux* in Act III, with Karen Kain and Frank Augustyn. (Track it down on video, if you can: it's a lovely six minutes of dance.)

This "rendering" of *School Education* is, so to speak, the Nureyev re-interpretation of the old ballet. And, like *Sleeping Beauty*, what comes at the beginning of the book may be somewhat puzzling. The fairies Authority and Docility arrive on stage, along with a number of philosophers and psychologists who have walk-on parts; and all the while we're waiting to get to the more interesting or practical bits. However, like *Sleeping Beauty*, these beginnings are foundational to the rest of the story; one might even say *vital*. Because understanding not only the "why" but the "Who" behind Non-Arbitrary Authority opens our journey into Relationship, and into "Affinities"; and these, in turn, begin to suggest a Curriculum.

You may, of course, single out something of delight or ornament, a particular *pas de deux* that matches your own needs or situation. But I hope that this story can also be viewed as a whole, with a message that builds throughout the various scenes.

"Education is an atmosphere, a discipline, and a life."

A Few Explanations

Why this book?

Because *School Education* is not just about school education. It starts with authority, and ends with a cooking lesson. But there's a lot more in between.

Did you use Charlotte Mason's own words?

In many places, yes. This is a re-presentation, not a paraphrase. However, some changes were made to amplify an unusual word, cite a source (including Scripture passages), or make a point sound more conversational.

Did you add other things?

Yes. But the intent was to remain as faithful as possible to the spirit of *School Education.*

Why did you re-order some of the chapters? Wasn't the original order important?

The order is slightly different. But as the students discovered, there's more than one way to bake little cakes.

The spelling in this book is inconsistent.

In most instances, the book uses North American spellings (with a Canadian flavour). However, in poetry and other word-for-word quotations, I have kept the original spelling and punctuation.

Who are these other people in the story?

Although the names may sound familiar, the characters are fictional, including Miss Mason's relatives.

Revitalized

An Educational Manifesto

"Studies serve for Delight, for Ornament, and for Ability."

Every child has a right of entry to several [i.e. various] fields of knowledge.
Every normal child has an appetite for such knowledge.
This appetite or desire for knowledge is a sufficient stimulus for all school work, if the knowledge be fitly given.

There are four means of destroying the desire for knowledge:—
(a) Too many oral lessons, which offer knowledge in a diluted form, and do not leave the child free to deal with it.
(b) Lectures, for which a teacher collects, arranges, and illustrates matter from various sources; these often offer knowledge in too condensed and ready prepared a form.
(c) Text-books compressed and recompressed from the big book of the big man.
(d) The use of emulation and ambition as incentives to learning in place of the adequate desire for, and delight in, knowledge.

Children can be most fitly educated on *Things* and *Books*.

Things, e.g.—
i. Natural obstacles for physical contention, climbing, swimming, walking, etc.
ii. Material to work in—wood, leather, clay, etc.
iii. Natural objects *in situ* [in their own context]—birds, plants, streams, stones, etc.,
iv. Objects of art.
v. Scientific apparatus, etc.

The value of this education by *Things* is receiving wide recognition, but intellectual education to be derived from *Books* is still for the most part to seek. Every scholar of six years old and upwards should study with "delight" his own, *living*, books on every subject in a pretty wide curriculum. Children between six and eight must for the most part have their books read to them.

This plan has been tried with happy results for the last twelve years in many home schoolrooms, and some other schools. By means of the free use of books the mechanical difficulties of education—reading, spelling, composition, etc.—disappear, and studies prove themselves to be "for delight, for ornament, and for ability."

There is reason to believe that these principles are workable in all schools, Elementary and Secondary; and that they tend in the working to simplification, economy, and discipline.

Part One: The Authorized Guide to Authority

"A switch stings more at the time but the strap smarts longer, that's a fact."

"I shall not use anything of the sort. I'm not going to whip my pupils."

"Bless my soul," exclaimed Mr. Harrison in genuine astonishment, "how do you lay out to keep order then?"

"I shall govern by affection, Mr. Harrison."

"It won't do," said Mr. Harrison, "won't do at all, Anne. 'Spare the rod and spoil the child.' When I went to school the master whipped me regular every day because he said if I wasn't in mischief just then I was plotting it."

(L.M. Montgomery, *Anne of Avonlea*)

"When *I* use a word," Humpty Dumpty said in rather a scornful tone, "it means just what I choose it to mean—neither more nor less."

"The question is," said Alice, "whether you *can* make words mean so many different things."

"The question is," said Humpty Dumpty, "which is to be master—that's all." (Lewis Carroll, *Through the Looking-Glass*)

Study 1: In Which Miss Mason is Interviewed

School Education begins with two things: a discussion of the relationship between parents and children (noting how that had changed in Miss Mason's lifetime); and an examination of how we understand authority (and again, how that had changed). In a baby-with-bathwater philosophical shift, authority itself had become viewed as the villain, rather than just its misuses. But even "without" authority, relationships were still coming apart—just in new ways.

It is a spring day in 1904. We join a young journalist, Miss Hagan, in the Scale How sitting room of Charlotte Mason, the sixty-something director of the educational operations at Ambleside. Introductions have been made, and the tea has been poured.

Miss Mason: I understand that you wish to discuss our philosophy of education in schools. But before children go to school, or begin formal lessons, they begin their education as "persons" in the home; and so we must begin with the principle of authority, specifically that which is held by parents.

Miss Hagan: How would you define that authority?

Miss Mason: It is that aspect of love which parents present to their children. Parents know it is love, because to them it means continual self-denial, self-repression, self-sacrifice. Children recognize it as love, because to them it means quiet rest and joyfulness of heart.

Miss Hagan: Has our view of this shifted over the years?

Miss Mason: The heads of households, years ago, were as autocratic as the Czars. Children received everything at their hands, from bread and milk to mother's love, with more or less gratitude, but with invariable docility. Everything was decreed, and all decrees were final. Only the other day I heard of an instance, the recollection of which had survived for seventy years. A boy of twelve or thirteen had been out shooting rabbits. He came home in the early darkness of a bitterly cold winter evening. His father asked him by which gate he had entered the park. "By (such a) gate." "Did you shut it?" "I don't recollect." "Go and see"; and the boy went, though he was already tired out, and the gate in question was more than a mile from the house.

Miss Hagan: Such an incident would scarcely happen to-day; the boy would protest that he was tired and frozen, and suggest that a servant should be sent to shut the gate, if it was important that it should be shut at all.

Miss Mason: But most parents meant well by it, and believed that by teaching their children such reverence for authority they were only doing what was right. The father in the story I just told you was a kind father, whom his children loved and honoured;

but arbitrary rule and unquestioning obedience were the habits of the household.

Miss Hagan: What do you mean by "arbitrary?"

Miss Mason: Unpredictable; with rules made and commands given on the spot. Parents knew that they *must* govern, that it was their duty; and they chose, often, to sacrifice close relationships with their children for the sake of that commandment. It is far easier to govern from a height, as it were, than from the intimacy of close personal contact. But you cannot be quite frank and easy with beings who are obviously of a higher and of another order than yourself; at least, you cannot when you are a child.

Miss Hagan: Were all families like this?

Miss Mason: There were, of course, rebellious children in well-ordered homes, perhaps one in a score, or one in a hundred, but these were the open rebels who would, sooner or later, come to a bad end; so we were told and so we secretly believed. And there were "ill-guided" homes where the children did what was "right in their own eyes" (Prov. 21:2). Those will always exist so long as there are weak and indolent parents, unconcerned about their responsibilities. But the rule and tradition, in most middle-class homes, was that of well-ordered and governed childhood.

Miss Hagan: Was there any positive outcome from this autocratic and arbitrary age?

Miss Mason: Yes, of course. It turned out steadfast, capable, able, self-governed, gentle-mannered men and women. In our less hopeful moments, we wonder as we watch the children of our day whether they will prove as good stuff as their grandfathers and their fathers. Every biography of someone who made his or her mark during the first half of the nineteenth century is a case in point.

Miss Hagan: How have things changed as we have entered the twentieth century?

Miss Mason: The relations between children and parents, and indeed between children and their grown-up friends generally, are far more intimate, frank and friendly than such relations used to be. There does not seem to be any longer that great gulf fixed between child thought and grown-up thought, which the older ones among us once tried to cross with frantic but vain efforts. Children no longer feel they have to be reluctant to speak out, for instance about things they are afraid of, or to clarify misunderstandings. Just to know that they can ask and tell is a great outlet. It means, to the parent, the power of direction; and to the child, free and natural development.

Miss Hagan: So first we had autocracy, holding on too tightly to authority. Then we moved into denial of one's authority. And in both cases the mistake is compounded by…arbitrariness?

Miss Mason: Anyone under authority holds and fulfils a trust. A trust is something given by someone above oneself, correct?

Miss Hagan: Yes, of course.

Miss Mason: When a person governs upon the impulse of his own will…or, as I would prefer to say it, willfully, *without* following the Way of the Will at all… he ceases to be *author*itative and *author*ized, and becomes arbitrary and autocratic. Ebenezer Scrooge was right when he said that a blot of mustard or a crumb of cheese could affect the senses; and in the same way, if we are at the mercy of the arbitrary temper, the impulse of will, then any "slight disorder of the stomach makes it cheat."

And though we like to say now that we are no longer autocrats in the home or in the classroom, that we have friendlier relations nowadays, the authority we see is still, often, arbitrary, *because* we have lost our understanding of authority itself. Parents and teachers, because their subjects are so docile and so feeble, are tempted more than others to the arbitrary temper, to say—"Do thus and thus because I bid you." "Because I said so." "Because I will punish you." They rule by temper and by terror, because they are unsure of what authority may be behind them. But the confusion, in both extremes, came from a mistaken idea of the ultimate authority. That is, Authority, with the capital "A."

Miss Hagan: What do you mean by that?

[Miss Mason goes to the bookcase and pulls out first one book, then another.]

Miss Mason: *(Putting a book down on the table)* First, John Locke, the great Enlightenment philosopher and the "father of liberalism."

Miss Hagan: What has he to do with the relationship between parents and children?

Miss Mason: A great deal. Two centuries ago, Locke promoted the doctrine of the infallible reason. That was, that we must do all our learning for ourselves, based on what we see and experience, and on our own mind's reflection about those things. When we accept that doctrine, individual reason becomes the ultimate authority, and every man is free to do that which is right in his own eyes.

Now we need to understand one thing about what Locke meant, a special limitation, if you will: he was referring to reason that was fully trained, and the mind instructed as to the merits of the particular case; but such *proviso* was readily lost sight of, and only the broad principle remained.

Miss Hagan: You're saying that most people missed the part about having to *train* the reason, and just assumed that it was set up to function, without having to work particularly at it. But I'm a little confused: Locke lived in the seventeenth century, and we have been talking about a style of parenting that lasted well into the nineteenth. Are you saying his ideas did or didn't influence English family life?

Miss Mason: They were somewhat too radical for England, at least at the start. Our strong religious beliefs seemed to safeguard us from following Locke's ideas too closely. But when his writings jumped the Channel into France, there was a soil well prepared for the seed. Locke was eagerly read there because his opinions "jumped" with the thought of the hour. His principles were put into practice, his conclusions worked out to the bitter end; and thoughtful writers consider that this religious and cultivated English gentleman cannot be exonerated from his share of the guilt for the atrocities of the French Revolution.

Miss Hagan: But we're still only up to the end of the eighteenth century.

Miss Mason: Correct; but then we have our own, perhaps greater, philosopher, who carried the teaching of Locke to the inevitable conclusions which the earlier thinker shirked: Mr. Herbert Spencer. *[She points to the book containing Spencer's essays on education, published in 1861.]*

Miss Hagan: Herbert Spencer? Didn't he coin the phrase "survival of the fittest?"

Miss Mason: Yes, unfortunately. Parents still buy this little book, and they find it quite easy reading. They accept the philosopher's teaching when he bids them bring up children without authority in order to give them free room for self-development. But they do so without perceiving that it was the labour of Spencer's life to *eliminate the idea of authority* from the universe; that, by making these recommendations, he repudiates the authority of parents because it is a link in the chain which binds the universe to God. For it is indeed true that none of us has a right to exercise authority, in things great or small, except as we are, and acknowledge ourselves to be, deputed by the one supreme and ultimate Authority. Instead, Spencer proclaimed, as they did in revolutionary France, the culmination–even the *deification*–of Reason.

Miss Hagan: Can you give me an example?

Miss Mason: One of Spencer's essays is titled "What Knowledge is of Most Worth?" His conclusion was that the knowledge of science was most important; and if we act on that principle, the content and manner of our teaching will reflect that. For instance, the application of scientific principles to homemaking has improved families' hygiene, nutrition, and so forth. This book was, indisputably, a valuable contribution to educational thought, and even practical life. But many people read it and embrace it, as a whole, without seeing that it is just one part of an entire philosophy, and if they were more aware of that whole, they might have second thoughts about Spencer's ideas on child-rearing and education. He would not have children do as they are bid, lest they should learn, as adults, to obey that Authority which we believe to be Divine.

[Miss Mason opens a third book, the Poems of Jean Ingelow.*]*

By this process of exhaustive reason, Spencer concludes, that, as this poet says—

> "We sit unowned upon our burial sod,
> And know not whence we come nor whose we be."

Miss Hagan: So God is dead, or at least has no authority over us. And the next logical step after that is…

[There is a knock at the door, and Miss Mason is called to deal with a college issue.]

Poetic Interlude #1

Miss Hagan remains at the tea table, leafing through the books. She reads more of Ingelow's poem "Honours—Part II," which is about a scholar musing on the true meaning of academic success.

O God, O kinsman loved, but not enough!
O man, with eyes majestic after death,
Whose feet have toiled along our pathways rough,
Whose lips drawn human breath!

By that one likeness which is ours and Thine,
By that one nature which doth hold us kin,
By that high heaven where, sinless, Thou dost shine
To draw us sinners in,

By Thy last silence in the judgment-hall,
By long foreknowledge of the deadly tree,
By darkness, by the wormwood and the gall,
I pray Thee visit me...

Come, lest this heart should, cold and cast away,
Die ere the guest adored she entertain—
Lest eyes which never saw Thine earthly day
Should miss Thy heavenly reign.

Are there no briers across Thy pathway thrust?
 Are there no thorns that compass it about?
Nor any stones that Thou wilt deign to trust
  My hands to gather out?

O if Thou wilt, and if such bliss might be,
 It were a cure for doubt, regret, delay—
Let my lost pathway go—what aileth me?—
  There is a better way.

What though unmarked the happy workman toil,
 And break unthanked of man the stubborn clod?
It is enough, for sacred is the soil,
  Dear are the hills of God.

Far better in its place the lowliest bird
 Should sing aright to Him the lowliest song,
Than that a seraph strayed should take the word
  And sing His glory wrong.

Friend, it is time to work. I say to thee,
 Thou dost all earthly good by much excel;
Thou and God's blessing are enough for me:
  My work, my work—farewell!

Study 2: The Interview Continues

[Miss Mason has returned to the table, and picks up immediately on the question that was left hanging.]

Miss Mason: From the dethronement of the divine, follows the dethronement of all human authority, whether it be of kings and their deputies over nations, or of parents over families. "Every act of authority is (*we are told*) an infringement of the rights of man or of child." "Children are to be brought up from the first self-directed, doing that which is right in their own eyes, governed by the reason which is to be trained, by experience of right and wrong, in the choosing of the right course." "Life has its penalties for those who transgress the laws of reason, and the child should be permitted to learn these laws through the intervention of these penalties." But "thou shalt" and "thou shalt not" are to be eliminated from the vocabulary of parents.

So complete and detailed is Mr. Spencer's scheme for the emancipation of children from rule, that he objects to the study of languages on the ground that the rules of grammar are a transgression of the principle of liberty. But consider this example, from our own school, of an oral lesson in grammar *[Appendix A]*.

Miss Hagan: Subject, English Grammar. Group, Language. Class II. Average age, 10. Time, 20 minutes.

Miss Mason: Note the objectives of the lesson.

Miss Hagan: One, to increase the children's power of reasoning and attention. Two, to increase their knowledge of English Grammar. Three, to introduce a new part of speech—preposition.

Miss Mason: So in one twenty-minute lesson on prepositions, we aim to give children not only more *power* over their abilities to reason and to pay close attention, but also more *knowledge*, and to open one more small door into the understanding of our language, that may help them as well when they learn the grammar of other languages.

We even give them the bonus of a Latin prefix: "Because these little words always take objects after them, and because their place is before the object, they are called prepositions, "pre" being the Latin word for "before," and "position" another word for 'place."' Does it seem to you that we would do children any favour by "emancipating" them from such knowledge?

Miss Hagan: But as you have said yourself elsewhere, the belief that you have only yourself to obey is, essentially, false. For example, children in a progressive classroom may be told that there are no rules; but when a fight breaks out, the teacher will probably come down hard on them, harder even than is reasonable. Such as punishing the whole class for a few children's misbehaviour.

Miss Mason: The arbitrary side of authority, yes.

Miss Hagan: Or something like the French Revolution, where everyone was shouting about personal liberty—but there were still people directing the drama. Is that what you mean?

Miss Mason: Yes, perhaps. The abuse of authority gives us the slave and the despot; but slavery and despotism could not exist except that they are founded upon elemental principles in human nature. We all have it in us to serve or to rule as occasion demands. To dream of liberty, in the sense of every man his own sole governor, is as futile as to dream of a world in which apples do not necessarily drop from the tree, but may fly off at a tangent in any direction.

But here is a greater problem: the influence of Spencer's rationalistic philosophy is by no means confined to those who have read his great works, or even to those who have actually *read* his essays on education. There is hardly a home, of even the lowest stage of culture, where his theory of education has not been either consciously adopted *or* rejected, even though the particular parents in question may never have heard of the philosopher. In other words, those ideas started to move and they did not stop. An idea, once launched, is "in the air," so we say. As is said of the Holy Spirit, we know not whence it comes, nor whither it goes.

Miss Hagan: Whether we're talking about Locke, or Spencer, or some other writer, it can be a hard job to have to examine every principle that presents itself. Does that mean we should avoid reading these books?

Miss Mason: Not at all. Perhaps even a work based on an erroneous idea may hold an important truth, if we can read with discernment. For instance, we ask "What is Authority?" The question itself shows us how inevitable in the evolution of thought has been the work of the rationalistic philosophers. It is to them we owe our deliverance from the autocrat, whether on the throne or in the family.

Miss Hagan: So if you were trying to un-make what the rationalists created, or to undo the damage they caused, where would you start?

Miss Mason: People have become weary of themselves. The notion of the finality of human reason has grown an intolerable limitation. Nothing less than the Infinite will satisfy the spirit of a person. We again recognize that we are made for God, and have no rest until we find Him; and philosophic thought, at home and abroad, has, to some degree, left these channels high and dry, and is running in other courses, towards the Infinite and the Divine.

We need to restore Authority to its ancient place as an ultimate fact, no more to be accounted for than is the principle of gravitation, and as binding and universal in the moral world as is that other principle in the natural. Fitting in to that of authority, as the ball fits the socket to make a working joint, is the other universal and elemental principle of Docility, and upon these two hang all possibilities of law and order, government and progress.

Miss Hagan: As you said, Spencer's book has influenced education for the past fifty years. But now that we're in the twentieth century, do you think it's time for the gate to swing the other way?

Miss Mason: It would seem to be thus that God educates the world. A philosopher sees that some principle is truth; it takes possession of him and he believes it to be the *whole* truth, and urges it to the point of *reductio ad absurdum*. Then the principle at the opposite pole of thought is similarly illuminated and glorified by a succeeding school of thought; and, later, it is discerned that it is not by either principle, but by *both*, that we live. So it seems not impossible that this century may see the advent of a truly great philosopher, who shall not be confined by the limitations of rationalistic or of materialistic thought.

Miss Hagan: Do you have one particular thinker in mind?

[Miss Mason pulls another book from the pile]

Miss Mason: Ten years ago, this volume on *Social Evolution* was published by Mr. Benjamin Kidd, who is known for his work in the area of sociology. The book has already done much for the recognition of these two fundamental principles. Why a football team should obey its captain, an army its commanding officer; why a street crowd should stand in awe of two or three policemen; why property should be respected, when it is the many who want and the few who have; why, in a word, there should be rule and not anarchy in the world—these are the sorts of questions Mr. Kidd sets himself to answer.

Miss Hagan: I'm familiar with that book. But doesn't Benjamin Kidd promote Darwinism as much as Herbert Spencer?

Miss Mason: What I have found interesting in *Social Evolution* is, as I said, the study of how authority and docility work, and perhaps the admission that they do exist and hold a place in our society; rather than a rationalistic attempt to explain *why* they exist.
Let me now ask you a few questions.

Miss Hagan: All right.

Miss Mason: Is every human soul born free?

Miss Hagan: That depends on what we mean by free.

Miss Mason: Is liberty our unalienable right?

Miss Hagan: Again, we would have to define liberty. But I would say, yes, most people today think they have a right to be "free," even if they're not quite sure what that means, or how other people's "freedom" affects their own.

Miss Mason: Is an offense against the liberty of a human being a capital offense?

Miss Hagan: Such as…kidnapping them?

Miss Mason: What about lesser "offenses against liberty" such as insisting that children go to church? Or requiring students to do arithmetic? Or asking employees to do tasks they dislike?

Miss Hagan: I think liberty gets a bit tangled there with rightful authority, or doing what you have agreed to do or you know you are supposed to do (which I assume is how you define docility).

Miss Mason: These are the same three questions that the rationalistic philosophers posed, that shook the earth in France, and that later began to be asked here as well. Before that time, we believed that authority was vested in persons, that arbitrary action became such persons, and that slavish obedience was good for the others. We believed in the "divine right" of kings and of parents, because we believed that the very will of God was an arbitrary will. But now we have been taught better; we know now that authority is vested in the office and not in the person; that the moment it is treated as a personal attribute it is forfeited. The person who is vested with authority requires no rigours of the law to bolster him up, because authority is not only *over* him, but *behind* him; and, *before* him is the corresponding principle of docility.

Even the rationalistic philosophers, like Locke, could not always take questions about authority to their inevitable conclusions without finding themselves in a mess of contradictions. But their important contribution has been, simply, to ask the questions.

[The interview is now at an end as Miss Mason prepares to take her daily carriage ride; but Miss Hagan arranges to come back on another day to discuss in detail what the PNEU students do in school. In the meantime, Miss Mason gives her copies of three articles she has (coincidentally) written on the topic of authority.]

Study 3: Authority and Habit

It sometimes happens that children, and not their parents, have right on their side: a claim may be made or an injunction resisted, and the children are in opposition to parent or teacher. It is well for the latter to get the habit of swiftly and imperceptibly reviewing the situation; possibly, the children may be in the right, and the parent may gather up his wits in time to yield the point graciously, and send the little rebels away in a glow of love and loyalty.

Nobody understood this better than the first Queen Elizabeth: it has been well said that she knew both when to yield and how to yield. Her adroitness in getting over many a dangerous crisis has been much praised by historians; but, possibly, this saving grace was not adroitness so much as the tact born of qualities proper to all who are set in authority. She had the meekness of one who has been given an appointed work, the readiness to take counsel with herself and with others, the perception that she existed for her people, and the quick and tender open-minded sympathy which enabled her to see their side of every question as well as her own—indeed, in preference to her own. These are the qualities proper to every ruler of a household, a school, or a kingdom. With these, parents will be able to order and control a fiery young brood full of energy and vitality, as Elizabeth was able to manage the kingdom when the minds of men were in a ferment of new thought, and life was intoxicating in the delightfulness of the possibilities it offered.

It is a little difficult to draw the line between mechanical and reasonable obedience. "I teach my children obedience by the time they are one year old," the writer heard a very successful mother remark; and, indeed, that is the age at which to begin to *give* children the ease and comfort of the habit of obeying lawful authority.

Authority in the Gospels

The centurion in Matthew 8 says: "I also am a man set under authority, having under me soldiers, and I say unto one, 'Go,' and he goeth; another, 'Come,' and he cometh; and to my servant, 'Do this,' and he doeth it." Here we have the powers and the limitations of authority. The centurion is set under authority, or, as we say, authorized, and, for that reason, he is able to say to one, "go," to another, "come," and to a third, "do this," in the calm certainty that all will be done as he says, because he holds his position *for this very purpose*—to secure that such and such things shall be accomplished. He himself is a servant with definite tasks, though they are the tasks of authority.

This, too, is the position that our Lord assumes; He says: "I came not to do mine own will, but the will of Him that sent me." That is His commission and the standing order of His life, and for this reason He spoke as one having authority, knowing Himself to be commissioned and supported.

Which is Which?

Authority is neither harsh nor indulgent. She is gentle and easy to be entreated in all matters immaterial, just because she is immovable in matters of real importance; for these, there is always a fixed principle. It does not, for example, rest with parents and teachers to dally with questions affecting either the health or the duty of their children. They have no authority to allow to children in indulgences—in too many sweets, for example—or in habits which are prejudicial to health; nor to let them off from any plain duty of obedience, courtesy, reverence, or work. Authority is alert; she knows all that is going on and is aware of tendencies. She fulfils the apostolic precept in Romans 12:8— "He that ruleth, [let him do it] with diligence."

But she is strong enough to fulfil that other precept from the same verse: "He that sheweth mercy, (let him do it) with cheerfulness." Timely clemency, timely yielding, is a great secret of strong government.

The Habit of Authority

We know Mr. Huxley's story of the retired soldier who was carrying home his Sunday dinner from the bakehouse (do older readers recall this once-common practice?). Some joker passed by who recognized the man's soldierly gait. "Attention!" he cried, and the man stood at attention while his mutton and potatoes rolled in the gutter.

Now, this kind of obedience is a mere question of nerves and muscles, a habit of the brain tissue with which the moral consciousness has nothing to do. It is somewhat the fashion to undervalue any but reasonable obedience, as if we were creatures altogether of mind and spirit, or creatures whose bodies answer as readily to the ruling of the spirit as does the ship to the helm. We think we have more power over our bodies than we really do: that we can make ourselves do what is right, by sheer willpower. (St. Paul said the same in Romans 7.) But, alas for our weakness! this description fits us only in proportion as our bodies have been trained to the discipline of unthinking mechanical obedience. We know the child who is fully willing to do the right thing so far as mind is concerned, but with whom bodily *vis inertiae* is strong enough to resist a very torrent of good intentions and good resolutions; and if we wish children to be able, when they grow up, to "keep under their bodies and bring them into subjection" (1 Corinthians 9:27), we must do this *for* them in their earlier years.

[What is ***vis inertiae****? The natural resistance of matter to any force acting on it. The harder you push me to do something, the more I don't want to do it.]*

Do we agree, first, that the response of docility to authority is a natural function? Well, then, the purpose of the daily routine of "small obediences" is to help children fulfill that natural function; to teach them to get their bodies to obey their own wills, by first training them to obey ours—with a non-arbitrary, non-autocratic way of authority.

It may be said that a child who has acquired the habit of involuntary obedience has proportionately lost power as a free moral agent; but, as the acts of obedience in question are very commonly connected with some physical effort, as, "Make haste back," "Sit straight," "Button your boots quickly,"—they belong to the same educational province as gymnastic exercises, the object of which is the masterly use of the body as a machine capable of many operations. (I am, I *can*.)

Now, to work a machine such as a typewriter or a bicycle, one must, before all things, have practice. One must have got into the way of working it involuntarily, without giving any thought to the matter. And to give a child this power over himself–first in response to the will of another, later, in response to his own–is to make a man of him. *["Man" meaning a person of integrity and honour.]* The failures in life are not the people who lack good intentions; they are those whose physical nature has not acquired the habit of prompt and involuntary obedience. The person who can make him/herself do what he wills has the world before him/her, and it rests with parents to give their children this self-compelling power as a mere matter of habit.

But is it not better and higher, it may be asked, to train children to act always in response to the *divine* mandate as it makes itself heard through the voice of conscience? Does it seem that we are less in contact with our spiritual natures, or with God, if we turn large parts of our lives over to habit? Should children not be taught early on to use their Will and Conscience in all things? Does developing that "self-compelling power" somehow lessen our acknowledgement that we are frail and sinful creatures in need of much grace and mercy?

The answer is, that in doing the first thing, we must not leave the other undone. There are few earnest parents who do not bring the power of conscience to bear on their children, and there are emergencies enough in the lives of young and old when we have to make a spiritual decision upon spiritual grounds—when it rests with us to choose the good and refuse the evil, consciously and voluntarily, because it is God's will that we should.

But it has been well said by a celebrated preacher that the effort of *decision* is the greatest effort of life. We find it so ourselves; shall we take this line of action or the other, shall we choose this or the other quality of carpet, send our boy to this or the other school? We all know that such questions are difficult to settle, and the wear and tear of nervous tissue the decision costs is evidenced often enough by the nervous headache it leaves behind. Now we must consider that this is even more difficult for the children. But with this wonderful provision in our tissues for recording repeated actions and reproducing them upon given *stimuli*—a means provided for easing the burden of life—it is startling and shocking that there are many children of thoughtful parents whose lives are spent in day-long efforts of decision upon matters which it is their parents' business to settle for them.

Consider the case of Maud. Her parents report that "Maud is too excitable, grows pale, acquires nervous tics." The doctor is consulted, and suspects that it is a case of over-pressure. Maud must do no lessons for six months; a change of air is advised, and she is put on a special diet. Somehow the prescription does not answer, the child's condition does not improve; but the parents are slow to perceive that it is not the soothing routine of lessons which is exhausting the little girl, but the fact that she goes through the labour of decision twenty times a day, and not only that, but the added fatigue of a contest with them to get her own way. Every point in the day's routine is discussed, nothing comes with the comforting ease of a matter of course; the child always prefers to do something else, and she usually does it. No wonder the poor little girl is worn out.

And then there is Louise, who seems born to be a lawyer and wants to know the "why" for every parental decision! It is not advisable to answer children too explicitly when they want to know the why for every command; but wise parents steer a middle course. They are careful to form habits upon which the routine of life runs easily, and, when the exceptional event requires a new regulation, they may make casual mention of their reasons for having so and so done; or, if this is not convenient and the case is a trying one, they give the children the reason for *all* obedience—"for this is right." In a word, authority avoids, so far as may be, giving cause of offence (2 Corinthians 6:3).

For all these reasons, we may quite *reverently* believe that we are so marvellously and mercifully made that most of our decisions arrive, so to speak, of themselves: that is, ninety-nine out of a hundred things we do, are done, well or ill, as mere matters of habit; and that we can also give that gift to our children.

Authority is Prevention, and sometimes Diversion

Another hint as to the fit use of parental authority may be gleaned from the methods employed in a well-governed state. The importance of *prevention* is fully recognized: police, army, navy, are largely preventive forces; and the home authority, too, does well to place its forces on the Alert Service. It is well to prepare for trying efforts: "We shall have time to finish this chapter before the clock strikes seven"; or, "We shall be able to get in one more round before bedtime." Nobody knows better than the wise parent the importance of giving a child time to collect him/herself for a decisive moment. This time should be spent in finishing some delightful occupation; every minute of idleness at these critical junctures goes to the setting up of the *vis inertiae*, most difficult to overcome because the child's will power is in abeyance. A little forethought is necessary to arrange that occupations do come to an end at the right moment; that bedtime does not arrive in the middle of a chapter, or at the most exciting moment of a game. In such an event authority, which looks before and after, might see its way to allow five minutes' grace, but would not feel itself empowered to allow a child to dawdle about indefinitely before saying good-night.

A good mother is the best home-ruler; she is in touch with the children, knows their unspoken schemes and half-formed desires, and where she cannot yield, she diverts; she does not crush with a sledge-hammer, an instrument of rule with which a child is somehow never very sympathetic. And we all know how important this, of changing children's thoughts, diverting, is in the formation of habit.

Perhaps the best aid to the maintenance of authority in the home is for those in authority to ask themselves daily that question which was put to our Lord— "Who gave Thee this authority?" (Mark 11:28). Let us not despise the day of small things (Zechariah 4:10) nor grow weary in well-doing (Galatians 6:9); if we have trained our children from their earliest years to prompt mechanical obedience, well and good; we reap our reward. If we have not, we must be content to lead by slow degrees, by ever-watchful efforts, to "the joy of self-control," the delight of proud chivalric obedience which will hail a command as an opportunity for service.

It is a happy thing that the "difficult" children who are the readiest to resist a direct command (those with the strongest *vis inertiae*?) are often the quickest to respond to the stimulus of an idea. The presentation of quickening ideas is itself a delicate art, which I have, however, considered elsewhere.

To conclude: authority is not only a gift, but a grace; and,

> As every rainbow hue is light,
> So every grace is love.
>
> (John Keble, *The Christian Year*)

Study 4: Liberty, not License

Masterly Inactivity

Are you yourself responsible, or accountable, for what you are? What you do?

It would be an interesting task for a literary expert to trace the stages of ethical thought marked by the uses, within living memory, of the word responsibility. Adults, and even children, were highly responsible years ago, but then it was for their own character, conduct, and demeanour. It is not at all certain that we hold ourselves responsible in this matter to the same degree. But we are apt to give ourselves more leeway in these matters than we allow to others. We are inclined to accept ourselves, instead, as inevitable, to make kindly allowance for our own little ways and little transgressions; and are, perhaps, wanting in that wholesome sense of humour, the gift of sufficient humility to see ourselves as we appear to others.

But there is another sort of responsibility that we should feel towards others, both near and far off. To those of us who believe we are all at school and have our lessons set as we are fit to take them in, this general sense of responsibility for others, a greater awareness of suffering and injustice, is an encouraging sign that we are being taught from above, and are, on the whole, "getting on." In other words, it is a good sign that we feel that anxiety for others' well-being.

And while we legitimately worry about the poor and the hungry and the unsaved, there is one more kind of responsibility which thoughtful people should take on themselves: parental responsibility. People feel that they can bring up their children to be something more than themselves, that they *ought* to do so, and that they *must*; and it is to this keen sense of higher parental duty that the Parents' Union owes its successful activity. But to perceive that there is much which we ought to do and not to know exactly what it is, nor how to do it, does not add to the pleasure of life or to ease in living. There is an uncomfortable stage between the development of this new power (knowing only that we want to do something differently) and the adjustment which comes with time and experience (others now approach *us* for advice).

The fundamental principles of docility and authority have been considered in the first place because they *are* fundamental; but, for that very reason, they should be present but not in evidence; we do not expose the foundations of our house. Not only so, but these principles must be conditioned by respect for the personality of children; and, in order to give children room for free development on the lines proper to them, it is well that parents and teachers should adopt an attitude of *masterly inactivity*.

But we must get clearly into our heads what we mean by that. The phrase comes from the writings of Thomas Carlyle, and means not interfering; but it has been misused to mean letting issues go unresolved, because we are afraid, or cannot be bothered, or feel overwhelmed. In any case, letting children or pets or the garden run wild for the sake of non-interference, is not the same as genuine *masterly inactivity*, or, as William Wordsworth put it, "wise passiveness." Masterly inactivity indicates that we have the power to act, the desire to act, *and* the insight and self-restraint which forbid action. If the distinction is still unclear, consider the garden: masterly inactivity does not allow plants to go to seed, or to be choked by weeds; but it also means that one doesn't pull them up every day to check on their growth.

We *ought* to do so much for our children, and are *able* to do so much for them (that sense of responsibility!), that we begin to think everything rests with *us*, and that we should never intermit for a moment our conscious action on the young minds and hearts about us. But that's when our endeavours become fussy and restless. We are "too much with" our children "late and soon" (to misquote Wordsworth). We try to dominate them too much, even when we fail to govern, and we are unable to perceive that wise and purposeful letting alone is the best part of education.

But again, this particular mistake arises from our legitimate concern and care for our children! So we may take heart: all that is needed now is *adjustment*; to this we must give our time and attention. A blessed thing in our mental constitution is, that once we receive an idea, it will work itself out, in thought and act, without much after-effort on our part; and, if we admit the idea of *masterly inactivity* as a factor in education, we shall find ourselves framing our dealings with children from this standpoint, without much conscious effort.

But there is, from our point of view at any rate, a further idea conveyed in masterly inactivity. The mastery is not over ourselves only; there is also a sense of authority, which our children should be as much aware of when it is inactive as when they are doing our bidding. I am not sure that without that our activities, or our inactivity, will produce any great results. This element of strength is the backbone of our position. The children understand that they are free under authority, which is liberty; but to be free without authority is license.

When the Child becomes the Autocrat

We must add a warning for adults who worry so much about seeming too autocratic that they become weak and refuse to assume their role and responsibility. The tendency to assume self-derived power is common to us all, even the meekest of us, and calls for special watchfulness; the more so, because it shows itself fully as often in remitting duties and in granting indulgences as in inflicting punishments. It is flattering when a child comes up in the winning, coaxing way those "monkeys" know how to assume, and says, "*Please* let me stay at home this morning, only this once!" This then changes to, "I don't want to go out," and, next, "I won't!" The parent who has no principle behind his own will soon learns that a child can be autocratic too—autocratic and belligerent to an alarming extent.

Fate and Freewill

This is the freedom which a child enjoys who has the confidence of his parents as to his comings and goings and childish doings, and who is all the time aware of their authority. He is brought up in the school proper for a being whose life is conditioned by "fate" and "freewill." He has liberty, that is, with a sense of must behind it to relieve him of that unrest which comes with the constant effort of decision. He is free to do as he ought, but knows quite well in his secret heart that he is not free to do that which he ought not.

The child who, on the contrary, grows up with no strong sense of authority behind his actions, but who receives many exhortations to "be good and obedient and whatnot," is aware that he may choose either good or evil; he may obey or not, he may tell the truth or not; and, even when he chooses aright, he does so at the cost of a great deal of nervous wear and tear. His parents have removed the support of their authority in the difficult choice of right-doing, and he is left alone to make that most trying of all efforts, the effort of decision.

Is the distinction between being free to choose the right at one's own option, and not free to do the wrong, too subtle to be grasped, too elusive to be practical? It may be so, but it is precisely the distinction which we are aware of in our own lives so far as we keep ourselves consciously under the divine governance. We are free to go in the ways of right living, and have the happy sense of liberty of choice, but the ways of transgressors are hard. We are aware of a restraining hand in the present, and of sure and certain retribution in the future.

Just this delicate poise is to be aimed at for the child. He must be treated with full confidence, and must feel that right-doing is his own free choice, which his parents trust him to make; but he must also be very well aware of the deterrent force in the background, watchful to hinder him when he would do wrong.

Study 5: Unproddable

Those Who are Prodded

Boys and girls are, on the whole, good, and desirous to do their duty. If we expect the "tale of bricks" (Exodus 5:18: *"tale" means quota*) to be delivered at the due moment without urging or entreating, rewarding or punishing, in nine cases out of ten we shall get what we look for. Where many of us err is in leaning too much to our own understanding and our own efforts, and not trusting sufficiently to the dutiful impulse which will carry children through the work they are expected to do.

One of the features, and one of the disastrous features, of modern society, is that we depend upon **prodders** and encourage a vast system of prodding.

> *[**Prodder:** A rod or pointed object used to poke or jab. Or, less literally, a person who tries to provoke an action or response from someone else. At its gentlest: the person who stands in the wings and prompts actors who have forgotten their lines, or who knocks on the dressing-room door to say "Five minutes, Mr. Olivier." At its other extreme: anything involving electricity.]*

We are prodded to our social duties, to our charitable duties, and to our religious duties. If we pay a subscription to a charity, we expect the secretary to prod us when it becomes due. If we attend a meeting, do we often do so of our own spontaneous will, or because somebody asks us to go, and reminds us half a dozen times of the day and the hour? Perhaps it is a result of the hurry of the age that there is a curious division of labour, and society falls into those who prod and those who are prodded.

Not that anybody prods in all directions, nor that anybody else offers himself entirely as a pincushion. It is more true, perhaps, to say that we all prod, and that we are all prodded. Now, an occasional pinprick is stimulating and wholesome, but the *vis inertiae* of human nature is such that we would rather lean up against a wall of spikes than not lean at all.

What we must guard against in the training of children is the danger of their getting into the habit of being prodded to every duty and every effort. School marks, prizes, and exhibitions, are all prods; and a system of prodding is apt to obscure the meaning of *must* and *ought* for the boy or girl who gets into the habit of mental and moral slouching against his prods. It would be better for boys and girls to suffer the consequences of not doing their work, now and then, than to do it because they are so urged and prodded on all hands they have no volition in the matter. The more we are prodded the lazier we get, and the less capable of the effort of will which should carry us *to*, and nearly carry us *through*, our tasks.

Only by masterly inactivity, "wise passiveness," or able "letting alone" can a child be trained "to reverence his conscience as his king" (Tennyson, *Idylls of the King*).

Notes for a New Era

> We all have it in us to serve or to rule as occasion demands. To dream of liberty, in the sense of every man his own sole governor, is as futile as to dream of a world in which apples do not necessarily drop from the tree, but may fly off at a tangent in any direction. (*School Education*, p. 10)
>
> "Chaos is dull; because in chaos the train might indeed go anywhere, to Baker Street, or to Bagdad [*sic*]. But man is a magician, and his whole magic is in this, that he does say Victoria [Station], and lo! it is Victoria..." (G.K. Chesterton, *The Man Who Was Thursday*)

How can you tell Autocracy from Authority?

If Autocracy is uneasy, Authority is:

If Autocracy is captious (petty, constantly fault-finding), Authority is:

If Autocracy is harsh one minute and indulgent the next, Authority is:

If Autocracy is self-sustained, Authority is:

If Autocracy is self-derived, Authority is:

If Autocracy is impatient and resentful, Authority is:

If Autocracy is swift to take offense, Authority is:

A Tool Kit for Masterly Inactivity

Here is the list of essentials (adapted from the chapter "Masterly Inactivity").

1. A sense of humour: frank, cordial, natural, good humour. This is quite a different thing from overmuch complacency, and a general giving-in to all the children's whims. The one is the outcome of strength, the other of weakness, and children are very quick to see the difference. "Oh, mother, may we go blackberrying this afternoon, instead of lessons?" The masterly and the abject "yes" are quite different notes. The first makes the holiday doubly a delight; the second produces a restless desire to gain some other easy victory (Mother's a pushover.)

2. Confidence. Have confidence in yourself as the parent (or teacher, or whatever situation you have been placed).The mere blessed fact of the parental relationship and of that authority which belongs to it, by right and by nature, acts upon the children as do sunshine and shower on a seed in good soil. And have confidence in the children. This is an element of *masterly inactivity* which I venture to propose to parents as a "blue teapot" for them "to live up to" (see the note below). Believe in the relation of parent and child, and trust the children to believe in it and fulfil it on their part. They will do so if they are not nagged or pestered about it.

   (What is a "blue teapot?" Some years earlier, Oscar Wilde had become famous for writing, "'I find it harder and harder every day to live up to my blue china." This was satirized in cartoons, and it seems to have become a common phrase by the era of *School Education*. In fact, Miss Mason's biographer Essex Cholmondeley mentions that whichever student was the "senior monitress" at Ambleside was, perhaps symbolically, put in charge of an actual blue teapot.)

3. Extra footwear that doesn't say "mom," whether that's hiking boots, basketball shoes, or high heels. If mothers could learn to do for themselves what they do for their children when these are overdone, we should have happier households. Let the mother go out to play! If she would only have courage to let everything go when life becomes too tense, and just take a day, or half a day, out in the fields, or with a favourite book, or in a picture gallery looking long and well at just two or three pictures, *without the children*, life would go on far more happily.

   Is this a hard saying for mothers in these anxious and troubled days? It may be hard, but it is not unsympathetic. If you will allow a much-used example, think of Aunt Frances in *Understood Betsy*. Always there for her little foster-child, to the point of obsession...her reading is all about children, her anxious interest is all in doing things right...until circumstances separate them and Aunt Frances is forced to start living her own life. If our interests are only about the children, we may need to back off. Just a bit.

4. An extra set of eyes for the back of the head. And anywhere else that matters. Parents and teachers must, of course, be omniscient; their children expect this of them, and a mother or father who can be hoodwinked is a person easy to reckon with in the mind of even the best child. For children are always playing a game half of chance, half of skill; they are trying how far they can go, how much of the management of their own lives they can get for the taking, and how much they must leave in the hands of the stronger powers. Therefore the mother who is not "up to" children is at their mercy, and need expect no quarter. But she must see without watching, know without telling, be on the alert always, yet never obviously, fussily, so. This open-eyed attitude must be sphinxlike in its repose. The children must know themselves to be let alone, whether to do their own duty or to seek their own pleasure. The constraining power should be present, but passive, so that the child may not feel himself hemmed in without choice.

5. Chill pills (so to speak). "A sound mind in a sound body" is another factor. If the sound body is unattainable, at least get the sound mind. Let not the nervous, anxious, worried mother think this easy, happy relation with her children is for her. She may be the best mother in the world, but the thing that her children will get from her in these moods is a touch of her nervousness—most catching of complaints. She will find them fractious, rebellious, unmanageable, and will be slow to realize that it is her fault—not the fault of her act, but of her *state*.

6. A stopwatch that, often, doesn't seem to work. Sometimes events hurry us, and sometimes—is it not true?—we like the little excitement of a rush. The children like it, too, at first. Father's birthday is coming, and Nellie must recite a poem for him; the little celebration has only been thought of a week in advance, and Nellie is seized at all sorts of odd moments to have some lines of the recitation crammed into her. At first she is pleased and important, and goes joyously to the task; but by-and-by it irks her; she is cross and naughty, is reproached for want of love for father, sheds tears over her verses, and, though finally the little performance may be got through very well, Nellie has suffered physically and morally in doing what, if it had been thought of a month beforehand, would have been altogether wholesome and delightful. Still worse for the children is it when mother or teacher has a "busy" day. Friends are coming, or the family wardrobe for the summer must be seen to, or drawers and cupboards must be turned out, or an examination is at hand. Anyway, it is one of those fussy, busy days which we women rather delight in. We do more than we can ourselves, our nerves are "on end," what with the fatigue and what

with the little excitement, and everybody in the house or the school is uncomfortable. Again, the children "take advantage", or so we say—the real fact being that they have caught their mother's mood and are fretful and tiresome. Leisure for themselves, and a sense of leisure in those about them, is as necessary to children's wellbeing as it is to the strong and benign parental attitude of which I am speaking.

7. A painting of Mary the Mother of Jesus, perhaps bundled with a recording of Pachelbel's *Canon*. The Madonna, no matter out of whose canvas she looks at you, is always serene. This is a great truth, and we should do well to hang our walls with the Madonnas of all the early Masters if the lesson, taught through the eye, would reach with calming influence to the heart for both children and parents. The mother would be able to hold herself in "wise passiveness," and would not fret her children by continual interference, even of hand or eye—she would let them be.

8. A sturdy backpack to carry all this in. The burden of children's training must be borne by their parents alone. But let them bear it with easy grace and an erect carriage.

9. A security lock on the backpack. The responsibility is the parent's, not the child's. The girl of ten who wishes to know if her attainments are up to the average, or the boy who discusses his bad habits with you and the best way of curing them, is displeasing, because one feels instinctively that such a child is occupied with cares which belong to the parent only. That free-will of man, which has for ages challenged faithful souls who would prefer to be *compelled* into all righteousness and obedience, is after all a pattern for parents. The child who is good because he *must* be so, loses in power of initiative more than he gains in good behaviour. But every time a child feels that he chooses to obey of his own accord, his power of initiative is strengthened. When it does occur to a child to reflect on his behaviour, he should have that sense of liberty which makes good behaviour appear to him a matter of his preference and choice.

10. Other ingredients go to the making of the delectable compound we call *masterly inactivity*, but space will allow me to speak of only one more. That highest form of confidence, known to us as *faith*, is necessary to full repose of mind and manner. When we recognize that God does not make over the bringing up of children absolutely even to their parents, but that He works Himself, in ways which it must be our care not to hinder, in the training of every child, then we shall learn passiveness, humble and wise. We shall give children space to develop on the lines of their own characters in all right ways, and shall know how to intervene effectually to prevent those errors which, also, are proper to their individual characters.

What is *not* in the tool kit?

1. "The bearing-rein may not be used." For those who have not read *Black Beauty*, a bearing-rein is also called an overcheck or checkrein. It forces a horse to hold its head up high (giving it a particular *bearing*), and was used for the purpose of making carriage horses appear more stylish. Even in Miss Mason's time, its use was questioned, not only because it made breathing difficult, but because prolonged use could damage the horse's spine. Moral: it's better to teach children to hold their own heads up freely than it is to achieve the same result by force.

Rules for the Unprodded

After *Study 5*, "Unproddable," Miss Mason's text goes on to give several practical applications for parents. The following is an adaptation of that list.

1. **Children should Choose their own Friends.** With regard to the choice of friends and companions, again, we should train children so that we should be able to honour them with a generous confidence; and if we give them such confidence we shall find that they justify it. If Fred has made a companion of Harry Jones, and Harry is not a nice boy, Fred will find the fact out as soon as his mother if he is let alone, and will probably come for advice and help as to the best way of getting out of an intimacy which does not really please him. But if Harry is boycotted by the home authorities and made the object of various prohibitions and exclusions, then Fred, if he be a generous boy, will feel in honour bound to take his comrade's part, and an intimacy which might have been easily dropped becomes cemented.

   What about class differences, or race, or other things that might spark particular parental dislikes, such as the fact that Mother doesn't like the way the friend's mother dresses, or that Father was once bullied by the friend's father? Where does legitimate concern for friends being good influences cross with personal taste or history? And of course there are those children who seem fine, and whose parents and homes should be quite acceptable, but who turn out later to have been a terrible choice as friends.

   Children need to learn to be good friends to others, as well as to choose their special friends wisely...something that, as adults know, is easier said than done; and as parents we wish that we could somehow keep them safe from disappointments, heartbreak, and even worse trouble. Unfortunately, that is exactly the point: that while we may occasionally be consulted for advice, more often we need to stay out of it, because this is a place where children *must* learn to stand on their own feet. Miss Mason's advice on choosing and keeping friends, as given generally throughout her books, is that we can find many, many, examples in literature (starting with *Jemima Puddleduck*, and moving on to Jane Austen and Shakespeare). For some children, "literature" in that sense would also include other media, such as movies; but it does *not* mean a specially-written story about a child who disobeyed his parents by making a friend who then got him in trouble. This gradual, no-finger-pointing growth in discernment seems more palatable to children than sermons and specifics.

(**Important note to parents:** occasionally there are "states of emergency" when the parental veto must be brought in, sometimes without being able to fully explain why to the child; and in that case, a successful outcome is going to depend on the trust that has been already established.]

2. **Children Should be free to Spend their own Pocket-Money.** Here is another opportunity for initiative on the children's part, and for self-restraint on that of the parents. Like the general teaching about friendship vs. interference in existing relationships, "financial literacy" should not be confused with parental control over a child's spending, especially as children grow older. Of course teaching children about real-life economics and budgeting is a very good idea, not to mention issues of credit and debt. As Miss Mason says, there is "no doubt that parents who dole out weekly allowances and have never given their children any large thoughts about money—as to how the smallest income is divisible into the share that we give, and the share that we keep, and the share that we save for some object worth possessing, to be had, perhaps, after weeks or months of saving; as to the futility of buying that we may eat, an indulgence, that we should rarely allow ourselves, and never except for the pleasure of sharing with others; as to how it is worthwhile to think twice before making a purchase—such parents cannot expect their children to think of money in any light but as a means to self-indulgence."

   So we need to have many talks like these, and perhaps work through some resource material on the subject. But that should have no obvious and immediate bearing on the weekly pocket-money: that should be spent as the children like, they having been instructed as to how they should like to spend it. Elizabeth Enright's book *The Saturdays* is a classic example, as is Sydney Taylor's *All-of-a-Kind Family*, where the five girls are free to decide how they want to spend their after-lunch pennies: pickles? Roasted sweet potatoes? Candy? And each of these treats gets shared all around.

   *"Gee!" [said Rush]. "I wish I had enough money to go to Carnegie Hall and hear something good. Schnabel or somebody." "You got your allowance today," said Mona… "Fifty cents isn't enough," said Rush. "And besides I need some shoelaces and a new writing pad and I owe a dime to a guy at school." (*The Saturdays*)*

Still, as in *The Saturdays*, pocket-money (and money earned by babysitting or other jobs) should not be just "fun money" forever: it should include the shoelaces, writing pads, and dimes we owe, etc., until, finally, those who have arrived in their teens should be ready to be trusted with their own allowance for clothing and other personal expenses. "The parents who do not trust their young people in this matter, *after having trained them*, are hardly qualifying them to take their place in a world in which the wise, just, and generous spending of money is a great test of character."

Do you notice Miss Mason's principle there? Train them—then trust them. We all admire spontaneity, but this grace, even in children, is not an indigenous wild-flower. In so far as it is a grace, it is the result of training,—of pleasant talks upon the general principles of conduct, and wise "letting alone" as to the practice of these principles.

3. **Children Should form their own Opinions.** There are burning questions in the air, seething opinions in people's minds. As to religion, politics, science, literature, art, as regards every kind of social effort, we are all disposed to hold strenuous opinions. The person who has not kept himself in touch with the movement of the thought of the world in all these matters has little cause to pride himself.

   It is our duty to form opinions carefully, and to hold them tenaciously insofar as the original grounds of our conclusions remain unshaken. But what we have no right to do is to pass these opinions on to our children. We all know that nothing is easier than to make vehement partisans of young people, in any cause heartily adopted by their elders. But a reaction comes, and the swinging of the pendulum is apt to carry them to a point of thought painfully remote from our own. In religious matters, it is not at all uncommon for children to grow up and choose a church which is quite different from that of their parents; and that should not be a great problem, if their religious education began with solid principles which will carry through no matter in which denomination they find themselves. Again: train them, then trust them.

   And as for politics? "Children are far more likely to embrace the views of their parents, when they are ripe to form opinions, if these have not been forced upon them in early youth when their lack of knowledge and experience makes it impossible for them to form opinions at first hand."

Part Two: Thinking About Education

Let us not in such wise impoverish our lives and the lives of our children; for, to quote the golden words of Milton: "Books are not absolutely dead things, but do contain a potency of life in them to be as active as that soul was, whose progeny they are; nay, they do preserve, as in a vial, the purest efficacy and extraction of that living intellect that bred them. As good almost kill a man, as kill a good book; who kills a man kills a good reasonable creature, God's image; but he who destroys a good book, kills reason itself—kills the image of God, as it were, in the eye." (*School Education*, p. 181)

I shall touch later upon the burning question of a curriculum which shall furnish children, not with dry bones of fact, but with fact clothed upon with the living flesh, breathed into by the vital spirit of quickening ideas. (*School Education*, p. 124)

In vain, through every changeful year,
Did Nature lead him as before;
A primrose by a river's brim
A yellow primrose was to him,
And it was nothing more.

(William Wordsworth, "Peter Bell—A Tale")

Study 6: In Which Miss Mason Lectures the Student Teachers on "Psychology in Relation to Current Thought"

The teachers' training at the House of Education began as a one-year course, but by 1904 it had been extended to two years. Teachers (or governesses) in training attended lectures with Miss Mason and other instructors, and also taught classes at Fairfield, the small Practising School. A student from that time recalled, "The whole atmosphere of the house was so extraordinarily good—nothing ignoble seemed within its doors, and moreover the actual surroundings, the books, the pictures (reproductions of old masters), the simple furniture and the wild flowers for decoration everywhere were a revelation in themselves in those days when the world either lived in a crowd of ancestral treasures or in the unutterable hideousness of the Victorian Age when prosperity had to be apparent" (*The Story of Charlotte Mason*, pp. 73-74).

We join the junior class as they prepare to hear a lecture on the philosophy and psychology of education.

Miss Mason: If the end of the eighteenth and the end of the nineteenth centuries have one feature in common more than another, it is that, in both, education comes to the front as among the chief ends of man.

The eighteenth-century people had the best of it. They had clear oracles in their Locke and their Rousseau. They knew what they wanted to do, and they did it with charming enthusiasm. The period teems with memoirs; and it is very pleasant to read about the philosophically and consistently brought up children of the more thoughtful families. They had *convictions*, and they had the courage of those convictions.

We, at the end of the nineteenth and the beginning of the twentieth century, are less happy. A few decades ago we too were in a furor of joyous excitement about education. Educational "movements," schools, colleges, lectures, higher education for women, public day schools for girls, examination tests which should give assurance on every point, were multiplied all over the country, and all over the world. It was a forward movement which has brought us incalculable gains; and not the least of these gains is the fact that today we are dissatisfied, and depressed, and inclined to wonder whether we are not on the wrong tack.

[laughter]

I mean that quite seriously. If educational work of the best kind had not been going on amongst us for the last two or three decades, we should not have arrived at this "divine discontent." Our pretty general dissatisfaction with education, as it is, is a wholesome symptom, as it probably means that sounder theory and happier practice are on their way to us. All the same, it is pretty evident that the time has come when we must change our front. Now, elementary schools; now, girls' high schools; now, public schools; now, women's colleges, are pronounced to be, on the whole, a failure. They do a great deal, it is said, but is what they do worth doing? Is it, in fact, education?

The bolder sceptics go so far as to attack our ancient universities; but they, very likely, will weather the storm because of their very inertness, the *masterly inactivity*, let us call it, which their opponents abuse; the universities do a great deal of "letting-alone."

One thing we begin to see clearly, that the stream can rise no higher than its source; that sound theory must underlie successful work. We begin to suspect that we took up schemes and methods of education a little hastily, without considering what *philosophy* or, let us say, *psychology*, underlies those schemes and methods. But, alas, psychologies are many, and educational denominations are bitterly opposed to one another. We must feel our way to some test by which we can discern a working psychology for our own age; for, like all science, psychology is progressive. What worked even fifty years ago will not work to-day, and what fulfils our needs to-day will not serve fifty years hence; there is no last word to be said upon education.

At the same time, that there should be at least half a dozen systems in the field, no one of them entirely satisfactory even to the persons who adopt it, shows that we who practise education should at any rate attempt to know the requirements of a sound system of psychology. That system which shall be of use to practical people in giving purpose, unity and continuity to education, must satisfy the following demands:

1. It must be adequate, covering the whole nature of man and his relations with all that is other than himself.
2. It must be necessary: that is, no other equally adequate psychology should present itself.
3. It must touch at all points the living thought of the age. That is, it must not be a by-issue to be discussed by specialists at their leisure, but the intelligent "man in the street" should feel its movement to be in step with the two or three great ideas by which the world is just now being educated.

And what are those ideas?

First, the *sacredness of the person*. You all know this quite well, as it is our first principle of education. But it shows up just as clearly in the great popular interest in hearing stories not only about those of the higher classes, but touching those of many walks of life. The interviewer does more than satisfy vulgar curiosity; what he has to tell is equally welcome to us all, whether he interviews the step-scrubber, the fruit peddler, the man of the book-barrow, "Harry and Harriet" out for a holiday, an ambassador, an author, an artist, a royal personage; every detail that will help us to realize the personality of one or other is more than welcome. So, too, we love popular literature that gives everyday details about the people, any people, of any county in England or Scotland, or indeed of any country.

We set an enormous and, I think, an increasing value upon *persons*, and any system of psychology which is to appeal to us must bring the *person* to the fore. He may be influenced by this and that; but he, himself, the indefinable *person*, of whom we are sensible while he is yet in arms, and of whom we never finally lose sight, however he be marred by vice and misery, must play for himself the game of life, and shape for himself those influences of environment, education, and whatnot, that do their part to make him what he is. A system of psychology which gives us the *person* in this sort of relation to educational forces should become common property at once, because this is what every mother of a family, every teacher of a school, and every sort of director of men or women already knows about.

Second, *the evolution of the individual.* Please understand what I mean here by "evolution": as we search for a system of psychology that puts the person in the first place, recognizes his value and individuality, we also look for a theory or system with one practical aim: making the most of that person, intellectually, morally, physically; and we acknowledge that a person can develop, grow, *evolve*, in each one of those ways. Education cannot be merely about loading a person with information, or even giving him or her a package of skills and accomplishments: such things are merely external, like a coat of paint. We, rather, desire an education that shall be *assimilated,* that shall become part and parcel of the person; and the psychology which shows us how to educate our children in this vital way will meet our demands.

Third, *the solidarity of the race*: that is, the human race. Our sense of the *oneness of humanity* reaches across the present, into the remotest past, and, we hope, into the future as well. Is it too much to expect that psychology shall take cognizance of this great educational force as well as of the two others I have indicated?

I do not say that these three are the only, so to speak, driving ideas of our age; but I think they are the three of which we are most aware. I think, too, that any system of psychology which takes no cognizance of either, or of all of them, does not afford that basis for our educational theory and practice of which we are in search.

So let us consider now some three or four of the psychologies which are not necessarily from this present time, but which have the most widespread influence. We do not presume to do this as critics, rather as inheritors of others' labour, who take stock of our possessions in order that we may use them to the most advantage. We will consider them in light of the three current ideas which I have already outlined.

The first is John Locke and his "States of Consciousness." As you remember from your philosophy readings *[Study 1]*, Locke did not concern himself with the mind or soul of man, but what he called "states of consciousness." Ideas, images, were for him to be got only through the senses; we can know nothing but what we get hold of through our own senses, assimilated by our own understanding. As for choice and selection in these ideas and images, Locke gives a comprehensive counsel—he says that "what it becomes a gentleman to know" is the proper subject-matter for education. The "mind" appears to have little colour or character of its own, but has certain powers and activities for the employment of the ideas it receives; and to account for these, Locke invented the pestilent fallacy which has, perhaps, been more injurious than any other to the cause of education—the fallacy of the "faculties of the mind."

[Murmurs in the classroom: "Oh, the faculties."]

Now let us bring Locke up to the standard which we have erected, remembering always that our power to raise a higher standard is *due* to him and such as he—he has, in a sense, given us the measuring tool itself—but does his own theory measure up to it? I would, briefly, say it does not. There is no unity of an inspiring idea, no natural progress and continuity, no ennobling aim, in an education which stops at "the knowledge a gentleman should acquire and the accomplishments a gentleman should possess." The *person* hardly appears except in the way of the semi-mechanical activities of his so-called faculties; he is practically the resultant, the combined effect, of the images conveyed through his senses.

What about the *evolution* of the individual? The expansion of the individual in the directions proper to him has no place here; every man is shut tight, as it were, in his own skin, but is taught to behave himself becomingly within that limit.

And the *oneness of humanity?* That intellectual commerce of ideas whereby the dead yet speak their living thoughts in the work they have left us, and by which as by links of an endless chain all men are bound to each and all men influence each, has no place in a philosophy which teaches that a man can know only through his own understanding working upon the images he receives through his senses.

Insofar as we wish to attain to the possibilities of the hour, we must take farewell of Locke, though we do so with gratitude, and even with affection.

The second system of psychology to be considered is modern Physiological Psychology. This works more or less on the same basis as Locke, but it adds an illuminating knowledge of biology. Here, as with Locke, the "mind" is apprehended only as "states of consciousness"; the senses are the sole avenues of knowledge, which reaches the brain in the form of ideas or images. I hope you have all done your reading from Professor William James of Harvard University, whose wise and temperate treatment of the subject commands the respect and attention of even those who differ from him. After explaining that what goes on in our brains is physiological; that psychology is, essentially, a natural science, something we can dissect and study as we do other parts of the body, Professor James writes this apologetic little conclusion:

> When, then, we talk of psychology as a natural science we must not assume that that means a sort of psychology that stands at last on solid ground. It means just the reverse; it means a psychology particularly fragile and into which the waters of metaphysical criticism leak at every joint, a psychology all of whose elementary assumptions and data must be reconsidered in wider connections and translated into other terms.

Professor James does not assume he has found all the answers; he seems to say that his work has simply opened up many more questions. This is soothing, and we close his book with satisfaction; but the pity of it is that all the "new" psychologists are not so modest as the Professor, some of them are, may we venture to say so, not a little arrogant: what is more, the student who goes carefully through this text-book of psychology is only too likely to consider that the author has proved his case—that psychology *is* a "natural science," "and it is," like Peter Bell's primrose, "nothing more"—up to the hilt, and he is not likely to go through a process of reconversion because of a few passing thoughts on the last page.

So in asking our questions about the "new psychology," let us keep in mind that we are speaking both of Professor James, and of those of his colleagues and disciples who take him at his word in saying that one may not be anybody after all, but exist only in a momentary state of consciousness. What a dreary thought! Hope goes out of life, for there is nothing pleasant to look forward to. If something agreeable should happen next year, there is no *I, myself,* to enjoy it; only the "state of consciousness" of some moment to come.

Does this seem so far that this theory will align with our interests in the "person," the "evolution," the "oneness?" No? Well, certainly not the *person*, if all our personhood is merely a current state of consciousness. And where there are no *persons*, there is no possibility of that divine afflatus, or inspiration, which we call *enthusiasm*; for that recognition of another on a higher plane which we mean when we say "I believe in so and so," for that recognition of the divine Being which we call Faith. Faith goes where all is fortuitous, where things come together by chance; when other people and ourselves are, so to speak, the circumstances of the moment. Faith, so to speak, needs there to be an *us* there.

Without that recognition of *persons*, and the corresponding lack of faith in anything beyond ourselves, we become devitalized. Life is flat and grey. We throw desperate, if dull, energy into the task of the hour because we shall so, anyway, get rid of that hour; we are glad to be amused, but still more glad of the stimulus of feverish work; but the work, like ourselves, is devitalized, without living idea, without consecrating aim. Our manner becomes impassive, emotionless; our speech, caustic, bitter, destructive; our countenances, dreary and impenetrable. Yes, you may well say "oh dear." But this is the change that is passing over large numbers of the teaching profession, men and women of keen intelligence, who might well have been inspired by high ideals, quickened by noble enthusiasms, had they not imbibed this new educational "faith," or lack of it.

We give what we have, and only what we have. But if these young educators' own aspirations have been swallowed up by this blighting, damaging system of thought, what vital ideas do they have left to pass on to children under their care? At this point we have lost relationships with ourselves and with other people; and we have also lost the ability to catch hold of Faith in a divine Being: this does not hold out much hope as a workable system of thought for us.

We should do well to be aware of this grey cloud hanging over education, but we need not sit down under it ourselves. Referring back to our original questions, is this system of psychology *adequate*? No: even the best of their own prophets–Mr. James, for example–freely allow that there is more in man than this system has ever dreamt of. Is it *necessary*? No, for as we shall presently see, more than one other psychology accounts with greater, though never with complete, success for the phenomena which a human being presents. Third, is it *harmonious with the movement of the age*? Again, no, emphatically no. It effaces that *personality* which this age tends to exalt and magnify, and to regard with tender interest, under even sordid conditions. Our third idea of the age, the principle of *solidarity with the human race*, is also lost, and connections of social and family life loosened; for what binding tie can there be between beings whose entity *may* be no more than a state of consciousness?

No, I did not miss the second idea of our age—it is coming now, but I am sure you can see where it conflicts with our view of *persons*, or *personality*. Again, the *evolution* of the individual is checked at the point of mechanical perfection. Such a system *may* turn out good mathematicians and clear-headed scientists; but what place is there in it for the higher forces of humanity, aspiration, speculation, devotion?

In conclusion, let me say that we have reason to keep watch at the "place of the letting out of waters" (Prov. 17:14), that is, the psychology upon which our educational thought and action rest. There is much we can learn from current research. For instance, the science of *anthropometry*, measuring the physical traits of humans, has yielded fascinating results: researchers are able to predict a number of facts about a child, say, from the way in which he stretches out his arm. Psychologists are also able to help, often, in dealing with certain childhood weaknesses, such as fears. But the danger is that we should take a part for the whole and allow this "new psychology" to usurp the whole field of education.

Well, we are out of time, but we still have some other theories to discuss. As preparation for the next class, I would like you to choose one of these three educators: Pestalozzi, Froebel, and Herbart, and find out what you can about his system of thought. Consider: does it seem necessary? Adequate? Relevant to the ideas of our age? Come prepared to defend your position.

Study 7: In Which Miss Mason Lectures on Other Psychologies of Education

In this study, the class of student teachers meets again, and Miss Mason questions them on what they have learned of the "great educationalists."

Miss Mason: Miss Breckenridge, will you give us your opinion on the contributions of the "two apostles of educational thought," Pestalozzi and Froebel?

Miss Breckenridge: I would say they contributed an idea that school should be pleasant and enjoyable. They promoted what we may call the enthusiasm of childhood, joyous teaching, loving and lovable teachers, and happy school hours.

Miss Mason: It is indeed a system of psychology to which our indebtedness is great. But does that seem adequate as a basis for education? Consider Froebel's word *Kindergarten* itself, the metaphor of children as cherished plants in a cultured garden. Can we detect any source of weakness in that concept? Miss Glass?

Miss Glass: "Make children happy and they will be good," is absolutely true, but does that idea develop the opposite point, "Be good and you will be happy?"

Miss Mason: Ah, yes, we come to the definition of our poor English word "happy," which you will no doubt recall from your reading of Plutarch's *Life of Solon*, and the story of how King Croesus argued with Solon about whether a poor man could be happy—meaning, perhaps, something more like blessed or fortunate, as in the Beatitudes of our Lord. But for the purposes of this *critique* we must limit its meaning to the more obvious one of showing pleasure and contentment.

Miss Capehart: Must we, though? As Miss Glass said, isn't that actually the point we are trying to make? We ask, are the child-plants in that delightful child-garden *too* carefully tended? Is the environment too perfectly tempered? Is it not conceivable that the rough-and-tumble of a home environment should lend itself more to the dignity and self-dependence of the *person*, and to the *evolution* of individual character? I suppose we have all noticed that children show more keen intelligence and more independent thought in home-play and home-talk than one expects of the angelic little beings one sees at school.

Miss Bruce: Humph, not always so angelic.

Miss Glass: Well, perhaps that is partly the children's attempt to assert their individual characters? A few pickles to set off all the sweetness.

Miss Mason: I daresay you all know Fra Angelico's picture of *The Last Judgement*? There is a detail which shows a circle of little monks (become as little children) dancing round, hand-in-hand, with the angels on their way to Paradise. The little monks are obviously very happy and very good; but somehow one misses the force of personality; they do not look as if they were capable of striking out a line for themselves.

[laughter]

We see this as a danger in the Kindergarten classes as well. Kindergarten teachers are doing beautiful work; but many of them are hampered by that metaphor of the *plant*, which is exactly lacking in that element of *personality*, the cherishing and developing of which is a sacred and important part of education.

The philosophic German mind beheld in man a part of the *Cosmos*, which, like the rest, needed only to be placed in fit conditions to develop according to its nature. The weak point in the argument is that man would appear to fall under the laws of two universes, the material and the spiritual; and that to energize and resist and repel is the law of his being. It will be said that this need not apply to the child; that the struggle for existence may well begin *after* a happy childhood has been secured; but probably any sort of transition violates the principles of unity and continuity which should rule education. To put it another way, we should begin as we mean to go on.

Miss Laurio: I believe, though, that today's Kindergarten teachers are, perhaps, more apt to include modern practices in their classrooms, such as art expression that gives children more initiative.

Miss Mason: Quite true: no doubt all thoughtful teachers recognize in what direction the limitations—all men have their limitations—of their Founder lay, and their practices are levelled up to modern thought. But it is well for us all to remember our origins and our tendencies, that we may recognize and avoid our dangers.

We now turn to the psychology of Johann Friedrich Herbart, another German philosopher of the past century, contemporary with both Pestalozzi and Froebel during the best years of his life. His theory of man is wide as the poles apart from either of those we have already considered; and there is no denying that it affords a tempting working basis for education. Miss White, please give us a summary of Herbart's educational thought.

Miss White: Herbart believed that people fulfilled their true purpose in life only by becoming productive citizens. He stressed individual development, but also in relationship with society and its values. He believed that each child was full of potential, but that potential had to be shaped by education. He used a five-step methodology in the classroom, where a teacher would prepare a topic of interest to the children, present the topic to them, and then question them *inductively* on what they had learned, giving them examples that would suggest a general rule or principle. Then the teacher would *deductively* sum up what the children were supposed to have learned from the lesson, and relate it somehow to their daily lives.

Miss Mason: Miss Capehart, can you add anything to that?

Miss Capehart: Herbart spoke of what he called "apperception masses," meaning, we might say, the "lumps of knowledge" that a child had already gained on a particular topic. It was important to build on what was already known.

Miss Mason: Miss Laurio, anything else?

Miss Laurio: Herbart was one of the first to promote the use of living books in the classroom.

Miss Mason: As do we. In fact, much of what you have said so far is true of our

PNEU philosophy and practice. Should we then consider ourselves Herbartian educators? What else must we consider?

Miss Bruce: You asked us to examine each system of psychology in connection with the two or three great thoughts upon which, as you have said, the world is being educated.

Miss Mason: And…?

Miss Bruce: I'm not quite sure. From what we've read, Herbart does have respect for the individual. He talks about individual potential, so that would seem to fall in line with concern for the *evolution* of the person.

Miss Mason: We should perhaps clarify exactly what Herbart means when he speaks of the individual. He does allow for a soul, but then he says this:

> The soul has no capacity nor faculty whatever either to receive or to produce anything. It has originally neither ideas nor feelings nor desires. It knows nothing of itself and nothing of other things. Further, within it lie no forms of intuition or thought, no laws of willing and acting, nor any sort of predisposition, however remote, to all this.

So this uneducated, unshaped person seems to have no *personhood.* All our complex notions of intellect, will, feeling and so on, disappear.

But since we do have the power of reacting on an idea…that is to say, the "soul" itself is no longer quite as it was after it has thus reacted…we may be filled up with knowledge, and shaped into productive members of society. The soul is thrown open to ideas—a fair field and no favour; and *ideas*, each of them a living entity, according to the familiar Platonic notion, crowd and jostle one another for admission, and for the best places, and for the most important and valuable coalitions, once they have entered. They lie below the threshold watching a chance to slip in. They hurry to join their friends and allies upon admission, and they form themselves into powerful "apperception masses" which occupy a more or less permanent place in the soul. And the soul—what does it do? It is not evident otherwise than as it affords a stage for this drama of ideas; and the self, the soul or the *person*, however we choose to call him, is an effect and not a cause; a result, and not an original fact. There we see the problem.

Now, again, any philosopher who emphasizes the potency of ideas deserves some attention. And indeed, we can become most enthusiastic when first we read Herbart's theory, or, more likely read *about* it, as in the book by Sir John Adams which is on your list. We get glimpses of a perfect theory—how *our* function as teachers shall be to supply the child always with fit ideas, and with the *best* ideas; how *we* shall take care so to select and arrange these ideas that they shall naturally fly to one another and make strong apperception masses once they have got beyond the threshold in the child's soul. Miss Breckenridge, as a teacher following Herbart's pedagogical methods, how might you teach the idea of… *[looking around the room for an example, she holds up a history book]*…a "book?"

Miss Breckenridge: We could start by learning about what books are, what they look like, what they're made of, and we could put some history in there, talk about what books have looked like in history. We could compare the colours, shapes, and sizes of books; and we could make our own books, learn some book-binding techniques. And after that we could talk about what books are for, how people have used books. We could have a field trip to a bookstore or a library, or a printing-house. And then after that we would have to start to find out the things in books, from Bo-Peep to philosophy and poetry. A month! No, that's enough to cover a whole school education. "Books" are definitely too wide a topic.

Miss Mason: Let us narrow it down somewhat. An example of co-ordinated study was done publicly some time ago, in London, *apple* being the idea round which the "apperception mass" gathered. You can imagine the sort of things the children did: counted apples, read books about apples, made applesauce, drew apple trees: I need not elaborate. But here is the problem with elaborate "units of study": if one is to find the principles of unity and continuity in the ideas presented to the soul, this is all good and well. But if, as we believe, these principles must *emanate* from the soul, or *person* (him or herself), this tempting "unity" may result in the collection of a mass of scattered and unassimilated information. To put it in the vernacular, an undigested mess from our educational Smörgåsbord.

Miss Laurio: Miss Mason, are there better ways to co-ordinate some of the studies?

Miss Mason: We do co-ordinate certain subjects without any reference to the clash of ideas on the threshold or their combination into apperception masses; but solely with reference to the natural and inevitable co-ordination of certain subjects. Thus, in readings on the period of the Armada, we do not devote the arithmetic lessons to calculations as to the amount of food necessary to sustain the Spanish fleet, because this is an arbitrary and not an inherent connection; but we should read such history, travels, and literature as would make the Spanish Armada live in the mind.

I will attempt to demonstrate the difference between such a study, based on natural co-ordination, and one which is designed to bring the "apperception masses" together. Imagine that, as Herbart's theory says, our souls begin with no ideas of their own. They are quite empty.

[She produces two empty bowls from under the desk.]

Given two souls supplied with precisely the same ideas, in precisely the same order…like two mixing bowls supplied with the same ingredients, in the same order…and with no other ideas whatsoever (which, as Sir John Adams points out, is almost impossible to achieve in real life, but we are speaking theoretically): we get duplicates of the same person. Is that even possible? If so, it would demolish once and forever that great conception, the *solidarity of the human race.*

Miss White: Excuse me, Miss Mason, could you explain that a little more?

Miss Mason: The American poet Walt Whitman expresses one side of this intuition when he tells us how he conquers with every triumphant general, bleeds with every wounded soldier, shares the spring morning and the open road and the pride of the horses with every jolly waggoner—in fact, lives in all other lives that touch him anywhere, even in imagination. But if these people we imagine ourselves connected with, past and present, far and near, are, like ourselves, not truly persons in essence, but only empty bowls filled up according to a formula, there is no reason to do so!

Miss Glass: I think I understand: we want to find other people like ourselves, but not identical to ourselves.

Miss Mason: How does the Herbartian theory affect our sense of the sacredness of the person? As we have said, by this reasoning, the person *per se* does not exist; or if he does, he is the mere sport of the ideas which take possession of him, whatever they happen to be. As for the evolution of the individual, it is not the *person* himself, but any mass of ideas which possesses him, that expands. The person now appears to be no more than a sort of vessel of transport to carry ideas into their proper sphere of action. Herbartian psychology is rich in suggestion, but we cannot take it up as it stands without losing the educational value of the two or three leading principles which are, as we say, "in the air."

We have now examined briefly the three or four psychologies which hold, more or less, the field of educational thought. We see that each *advances* truth, but that neither expresses the *whole* truth even so far as to afford a working basis for educators.

So where might we go from here? We work on "by rule of thumb," using common sense, our own experience, or random suggestions from other teachers, writers, or trainers of puppies—which is like throwing ingredients into the bowl at random. Or we borrow a fragment here and a fragment there from the various psychologies, as the case appears to demand; but in that, we are like children with a hard sum, whose answer they know, and who try first division, then multiplication, then subtraction, to make it come right. It seems obvious that we must do better than that. What have we, of the PNEU, to bring forward in the way of a working psychology which shall meet the demands I have indicated? That will be the topic of our next session.

Study 8: In Which Miss Mason Introduces the PNEU Principles, Part One

What are the principles on which to base a truer concept of education? "In the first place," says Miss Mason, "we take children seriously as persons like ourselves, only more so; the first question that comes before us is—What do we understand by a person?"

Miss Mason: Let me try to set forth, though with diffidence, what we have done in the Parents' National Educational Union, knowing that no man and no society can say of educational truth, "This is mine and that is thine"; for all is common, and none of us can know how much he gives and how much he takes.

We do not claim to be philosophers; we are modest and practical people looking out for a secure basis for education. It is just possible that bringing unbiased minds and a few guiding principles to the task, we have, not joined the parts of the puzzle, but perceived dimly how an outline here and an outline there indicate, not so many separate psychologies, but shadowings forth of a coherent, living, educational *principle* destined to assume more and more clearness and fulness until it is revealed to us at last as the *educational gospel*, the discovery of which may be the destined reward and triumph of our age.

Recall that a workable psychology of education:

1. must be adequate, covering the whole nature of man and his relations with all that is other than himself
2. must be necessary: that is, no other equally adequate psychology should present itself, and
3. must touch at all points the living thought of the age.

For years we have worked definitely and consistently upon a psychology which appears to me to satisfy all three of these points. I will begin, however, at the end, by offering the proof of this method: the children themselves. How does one recognize a PNEU student? Children brought up on this theory of education, wherever we come across them, are curiously *vitalized*; not bored; not all alive in the playing-field but dull and inert in the schoolroom—even when it is that place proverbial for dullness, a home school-room taught by a governess.

There is *unity* in their lives; they are not two persons, one with their play-fellows and quite other with their teachers and elders; but frank, fresh, showing keen interest in whatever comes in their way.

Then, too, there is *continuity* in their education. Little children are always eager to know; but the desire for knowledge seldom survives two or three years of school-life. But these children begin on lines that go on from the first baby lessons, through boyhood, girlhood, womanhood, motherhood; there is no transition stage, but simple, natural, living progress.

But the claims I venture to make for these children must rest not only on the evidence of the few, but on the principles upon which we work.

In the first place, we take children seriously as persons like ourselves, only more so; therefore the first question that comes before us is—what do we *understand* by "a person?" We believe the thinking, invisible soul and acting, visible body to be one in so intimate a union that, as Mr. Browning writes, "Nor soul helps flesh more now than flesh helps soul." The countenance of our friend with the thousand delicate changes which express every nuance of feeling; the refinement, purpose, perception, power, revealed in his hand; the dear familiar carriage; these are all inseparable from our conception of the person; as in Browning's verse, one's physical being is deeply connected with the soul.

Whatever is advanced by the physiologist and the rational psychologist as to the functions of that most marvellous brain cortex, the seat of consciousness, as furnishing us with images and impulses, of the motor nerves as originating action, of the brain as the seat of habit; of the possibility of educating a child in all becoming habits of act, in all sweet habits of thought, by taking measures to secure that these habits become, as it were, a memory of the brain to be awakened by due stimuli—all these things we believe and receive; and we believe further that the possibility of a rational education rests upon this physiological basis, only fully discovered to us within the present generation. We want to educate the soul; and we have found a path to doing so, through the physical nature, because there is unity between them.

But is it enough to assume that all this delicate brain mechanism is controlled automatically? That seems inadequate; we want to say that the person should possess such vehicle of expression and medium of relation to the outer world. More than that, we believe that the whole person wills and thinks and feels; is always present, though not always aware of him/herself; is without parts or faculties; whatever he or she does, *he or she* does, all of him (or her), whether he takes a walk or she writes a book. Now we are speaking again about unity.

It is so much the habit to think of the person as a dual being, flesh and spirit, that it is necessary to clear our minds on this subject, especially as it applies to education. We need physical food, and also mental food; but that alone does not prove that we are two different sorts of beings. A person is no more composed of ideas, on the one hand, than he is of nervous and muscular tissues on the other. And think of this: pleasant and well-cooked food makes man of a cheerful countenance, and "wine gladdens the heart of man"; and we all know the spiritual refreshment of a needed meal. On the other hand, we all know the lackluster eye and pallid countenance of the well-fed ones who receive none of that other nutriment which we call ideas; quick and living thought is as necessary for the full and happy development of the body as it is for that of the soul. We therefore believe that our educational doctrine is *adequate*, for since the person includes both and is more than both the flesh and the spirit, we are following the progress of biological psychology with avidity, making use of every gain that presents itself, while following with equal care the advance of philosophic thought. And, if our educational creed is by no means conclusive, we think it is not narrow, because we have come across no problem of life or mind the solution of which is shut out from us by any dogma of ours.

We cannot say that our doctrine is *necessary*, but we do say that some educational theory which shall include the whole nature of man and the results of scientific research, in the same or a greater degree, is necessary. We find ourselves, too, in touch with those three great ideas which seem to me to be the schoolmasters of the world at the present moment. The *person* of the child is sacred to us; we do not swamp his individuality in his intelligence, in his conscience, or even in his soul; perhaps one should add to-day, or even in his physical development. The person is all these and more. We safeguard the initiative of the child and we realize that, in educational work, we must take a back seat; the teacher, even when the teacher is the parent, is not to be too much to the front. There is no more facile way of swamping character and individuality than by *personal* influence.

Now I am going to give you a key to the whole matter. I have had it printed on these cards, which you may find useful as bookmarkers—Miss Laurio, will you please pass them out?

> We consider that *education is the science of relations*, or, more fully, that education considers what relations are proper to a human being, and in what ways these various relations can best be established; that a human being comes into the world with capacity for many relations; and that we, for our part, have two chief concerns—first, to put him in the way of forming these relations by presenting the right idea at the right time, and by forming the right habit upon the right idea; and, secondly, by not getting in the way and so *preventing* the establishment of the very relations we seek to form.

What do we mean by *preventing*? Half the teaching one hears and sees is more or less obtrusive. Kindly obtrusive, but obtrusive just the same. The oral lesson and the lecture, with their accompanying notes, give very little scope for the establishment of relations with great minds and various minds. I have even known of teachers who have thought well to compose the songs and poems which their children use. Think of it! not even our poets are allowed to interpose between the poor child and the probably mediocre mind of the teacher.

The child who learns his science from a text-book, though he go to Nature for illustrations, and he who gets his information from object-lessons, has no chance of forming relations with things as they are, because his teacher makes him believe that to know *about* things is the same thing as knowing them personally; though to know *about* Prince Edward is by no means the same thing as knowing the boy-prince, and to know *about* Prince Edward Island is not the same thing as being there.

So we study, in many ways, the art of standing aside.

People sometimes write that the books set in our school constitute much of its usefulness; they do not always see that the choice of books, which implies the play of various able minds directly on the mind of the child, is a great part, but still only part, of that education which consists in the establishment of relations. The art of standing aside to let a child develop the relations proper to him is the fine art of education, when the educator perceives the two things he must do and how to do them. And the *evolution of the individual* is a natural sequence of the opening up of relations.

How we labour towards *the solidarity of the human race* I hope to show more fully later on. But, for example, we do not endeavour to give children outlines of ancient history, but to put them in living touch with a thinker who lived in those ancient days. We are not content that they should learn the history of their own country alone; some living idea of contemporaneous European history, anyway, we try to get in; and so that the history we teach may be the more living, we also include some of the literature of that period, and some of the best historical novels and poems that treat of the period; and so on with other subjects. (Of course history is not the only subject that can be made a little broader and deeper with the addition of literature!)

Well, there is nothing new in all this; but what we venture to claim is that our work is unified *and* vitalized by a comprehensive theory of education and a sound basis of psychology. As your response to this class, I would ask each of you to write a one-page paper demonstrating the same. These will be due at the next lecture.

> It is possible that what stirred inside her head at that moment was her brain, waking up. She was nine years old, and she was in the third A grade at school, but that was the first time she had ever had a whole thought of her very own. At home, Aunt Frances had always known exactly what she was doing, and had helped her over the hard places before she even knew they were there; and at school her teachers had been carefully trained to think faster than the scholars. Somebody had always been explaining things to Elizabeth Ann so industriously that she had never found out a single thing for herself before. This was a very small discovery, but an original one. Elizabeth Ann was as excited about it as a mother-bird over the first egg that hatches. (Dorothy Canfield Fisher, *Understood Betsy*)

Study 9: In Which Miss Mason Introduces the PNEU Principles, Part Two

"Now let me ask two questions, to which we seem to have but one answer. First, what is the basis of habit? And, second, how do ideas behave?"

Part One

Miss Mason: I have laid before you, as a working hypothesis, that human beings–and therefore, children–are homogeneous, spiritual beings invested with bodies–capable of responding to spiritual impulses, the organ by which they express themselves, the vehicle by which they receive impressions, and the medium by which they establish relations with what we call the material world; –that will, conscience, affection, reason, are not the various parts of a composite whole, but are different modes of action of each person.

What do we believe about their **capacities**? That they are capable of many relations and consequently of many modes of action; that, given the due relations, their power of expansion in these relations appears to be, not illimitable, but, so far as we know, as yet unlimited.

What do we know of their **limitations**? That, deprived of any or all of the relations proper to him, a human being has no power of self-development in these directions; though he would appear not to lose any of his capacity for these relations.

What do we then say of their **education**? Again, that any relation once initiated leaves, so to speak, an organic memory of itself in the nervous tissue of the brain; that in this physical registration of an experience or a thought, or of the memory of an experience or a thought, lies the possibility of habit; that some nine-tenths of our life run upon lines of habit; and that, therefore, in order to educate, we must know something of both the psychological and physiological history of a habit, how to initiate it and how to develop it; and, finally, that a human being under education has two functions—the formation of **habits** and the assimilation of **ideas**.

Physiologists and rational psychologists have made the basis of habit pretty plain to us. The nature, functions, and behaviour of ideas, and how ideas have power in their impact upon the cerebral hemisphere to make some sort of sensible impression—all this is matter as to which we are able only to make guesses at truth. But this need not dismay us, for such other ultimate facts as sleep and life and death are equally unexplained. In every department of science we are brought up before facts which we have to assume as the bases of our so-called science. Where a working hypothesis is necessary, we can only assume those bases that seem to us the most adequate and the most fruitful. Let us say, with Plato, that an idea is an entity, a live thing of the mind.

And where do those ideas originate?

Apparently no one has power to beget an idea by himself; it appears to be the offspring of two minds. So-and-so "put it in my head," we say, and that is the history of all ideas—the most simple and the most profound. But, once begotten, the idea seems to survive indefinitely. It is painted in a picture, written in a book, carved into a chair, or only spoken to someone who speaks it again, who speaks it again, who speaks it again, so that it goes on being spoken, for how long? Who knows! Nothing so strikes the student of history as the persistent way in which ideas recur, except the way in which they elude observation until occasion calls them forth.

Our natural progeny, the children we bring forth, may indeed die and be buried; but of this spiritual progeny of ideas, who may forecast the history or foretell the end? But, even further: may we hypothesize that, as an idea comes of the contact of two minds, the idea of another is no more than a *notion* to us until it has undergone a process of generation within us? For instance, I am standing here speaking to you today, and I hope that the ideas I am offering to you are worthwhile and *vital*; but until they act on the *materiel* of your own brain tissue, until they have actually generated within you, they are not quite alive. We recognize that different ideas appeal to different minds—not at all because the ideas themselves have an independent desire to club into Herbartian "apperception masses," but because certain persons have in themselves, by inheritance, may we assume (because we are certainly not empty bowls), that which is proper to attract certain ideas.

To illustrate invisible things by visible, let us suppose that the relation is something like that between the pollen and the ovule it is to fertilize. The ways of carrying the pollen are various, not to say indiscriminate, but there is nothing haphazard in the result. The right pollen goes to the right ovule and the plant bears seed after its kind; even so, the person brings forth ideas after his or her kind.

Miss Glass: How can something as purely spiritual as an idea make an impression on our actual brain substance, or change our physical being?

Miss Mason: We do not know. We have some little demonstration that it is so in the fact of the score of reflex actions by which we visibly respond to an idea that "strikes" us. The eye brightens, the pulse quickens, the colour rises, the whole person becomes vitalized, capable, strenuous, no longer weighed down by this clog of flesh. Do we need to be in physical contact with those who give us ideas? Or even to live in the same time? No, certainly not. Every human being has the power of communicating notions to other human beings; and, after he is dead, this power survives him in the work he has done and the words he has said. How illimitable is life!

And, even further, the divine Spirit has that same intimate power of corresponding with the human spirit; our understanding of that needs not to be urged, once we recognize ourselves as spiritual beings at all. Nor does this teeming population of ideas arise to us without order and without purpose beyond the scope of our busy efforts and intentions. It would seem as if a new human being came into the world with unlimited capacity for manifold relations, with a tendency to certain relations in preference to certain others, but with no degree of adaptation to these relations. To secure that adaptation and the expansion and activity of the person, along the lines of the relations most proper to him, is the *work of education*; to be accomplished by the two factors of *ideas* and *habits*. Samuel Taylor Coleridge spoke of "captain" ideas, and so we agree that every relationship must be initiated by its own "captain" idea, *then* sustained upon fitting *ideas*; and *finally* wrought into the material substance of the *person* by its proper *habits*. This is the field before us.

You should all write this down for future reference:

> Every habit we have formed has had its initial idea, and every idea we receive is able to initiate a habit of thought and of action.

Part Two

Miss Mason: Plainly we have not to develop the *person*; he is there already, with, possibly, every power that will serve him in his passage through life.

But if we are not required, and indeed, not able at all, to develop the *person* of the person, what, then, have we to do for him? Some day we shall be told that the very word "education" is a misnomer belonging to the stage of thought when the drawing forth of faculties was supposed to be a teacher's business. We shall have some fit new word meaning, perhaps, "applied wisdom," for wisdom is *the science of relations*, and the thing we have to do for a young human being is to put him in touch, so far as we can, with all the *relations* proper to him.

We begin to see light, both as to the lines upon which we should form habits and as to that much-vexed question—the subjects of instruction proper for children. We are no longer divided between the claims of the classical and the modern side. We no longer ask ourselves whether it is better to learn a few subjects "thoroughly," so we say, or to get a "smattering" of many. These questions are beside the mark.

In considering the relationships which we may initiate for a child, I will begin with what we shall probably be inclined to call the lowest rung of the ladder. We may believe that a person–I have a "baby person" in view–is put into this most delightful world for the express purpose of forming ties of intimacy, joy, association, and knowledge with the living and moving things that are therein, with what St. Francis would have called "his brother the mountain" and "his brother the ant" and "his brothers in the starry heavens." Fullness of living, joy in life, depend, far more than we know, upon the establishment of these relations. Is everyone clear on the subject matter at hand? Miss Breckenridge?

Miss Breckenridge: We want the child to build relationships with the things in nature, which would include the earth itself, plant and animal life, oceanography, and astronomy. So, all things that eventually fall under science, and the more physical parts of geography.

Miss Mason: And, as educators, what do we generally do with that? We consider the matter carefully; we say the boy will make a jumble of it if he is taught more than one or two sciences. We ask our friends "what sciences will tell best in examinations?" and "which are most easily learned?" We discover which are the *best* text-books in the *smallest* compass. The most economical, so to speak. The student learns up the text, listens to lectures, makes diagrams, watches demonstrations. Behold! he has "learned a science," and is able to produce facts and figures, for a time anyway, in connection with some one class of natural phenomena; but of tender intimacy with Nature herself he has acquired none.

I will now sketch what seems to me a better way.

1. **The Power of Recognition.**—The parents of an infant know that the first step in intimacy is recognition; and we should measure a child's education, not solely by his progress in the "three R's," but by the number of living and growing things he knows by look, name, and habitat. A six-year-old in our first form will note with eager interest the order of time in which the trees put on their leaves; will tell you whether to look in hedge, or meadow, or copse, for

eyebright, wood-sorrel, ground-ivy. He will not think that flowers were made to be plucked; but he will take his friends to see where the milk-wort grows, or the bog-bean, or the sweet-gale. The birds of the air are no longer casual; he soon knows when and where to expect the redstart and the meadow pipit. The water-skater and the dragon-fly are interesting and admired acquaintances. His eyes have sparkled at the beauty of crystals, and, though he may not have been able to find them *in situ*, he knows the look of the crystals of lime and quartz, and the lovely pink of felspar, and many more.

2. **Aesthetic Appreciation.**—Aesthetic appreciation follows close upon recognition, for does the child not try from very early days to catch the flower in its beauty of colour and grace of gesture, with his own paintbrush? The wise mother is careful to open her child's eyes to another kind of appreciation. She makes him look from a distance at a wild cherry-tree, or at a willow with its soft catkins, and she shows him that the picture on a Japanese screen has caught the very look of the thing—though when he comes to compare a single catkin or a single cherry blossom with those on the screen, there is no portraiture; and so he begins to learn at a very early age that to paint that which we *see*, and that which we *know to be there*, are two different things; and that the former art is the more gratifying.

3. **First-hand Knowledge.**—By-and-by he passes from acquaintance, the pleasant recognition of friendly faces, to knowledge, the sort of knowledge we call *science*. He begins to notice that there are resemblances between wild-rose and apple blossom, between buttercup and wood-anemone, between the large rhododendron blossom and the tiny heath floret. A suggestion will make him find out accurately what these resemblances are, and he gets the new and delightful idea of *families* of plants. His little bit of knowledge is real science, because he gets it at first-hand; in his small way he is another Carolus Linnæus, sorting and classifying the things he knows.

4. **Appreciative Knowledge and Exact Knowledge.**—All the time he is storing up associations of delight, which will come back for his refreshment when he is an old man. With this sort of appreciative knowledge of things to begin with, the superstructure of exact knowledge, living science, no mere affair of text-books and examinations, is easily raised, because a natural desire is implanted. We might say the same of art—that the child who has been taught to *see* appreciates pictures with discrimination.

And what sorts of sciences will this curriculum cover? Geology, mineralogy, physical geography, botany, natural history, biology, astronomy—the whole circle of the sciences is, as it were, set with gates ajar in order that a child may go forth furnished, not with scientific knowledge, but with what Thomas Huxley calls "common information," so that he may feel for objects on the earth and in the heavens the sort of proprietary interest which the son of an old house has in its heirlooms.

Miss Breckenridge, you look as if you had something to say.

Miss Breckenridge: Wasn't Huxley the one they called "Darwin's bulldog," and who coined the word "agnosticism?" It doesn't seem as if he'd have much to say to us.

Miss Mason: Sometimes we can find truth in unlikely places. Here is what Huxley wrote in the preface to his book *Physiography*:

> It appeared to me to be plainly dictated by common sense, that the teacher, who wishes to lead his pupil to form a clear mental picture of the order which pervades the multiform and endlessly shifting phenomena of nature, should commence with the familiar facts of the scholar's daily experience; and that, from the firm ground of such experience, he should lead the beginner, step by step, to remoter objects and to the less readily comprehensible relations of things.

Yes so far?

> In short, that the knowledge of the child should, of set purpose, be made to grow, in the same manner as that of the human race has spontaneously grown.
>
> I conceived that a vast amount of knowledge respecting natural phenomena and their interdependence, and even some practical experience of scientific method, could be conveyed, with all the precision of statement, which is what distinguishes science from common information; and, yet, without overstepping the comprehension of learners who possessed no further share of preliminary educational discipline, than that which falls to the lot of the boys and girls who pass through an ordinary primary school. And I thought, that, if my plan could be properly carried out, it would not only yield results of value in themselves, but would facilitate the subsequent entrance of the learners into the portals of the special sciences.

And just afterwards, he adds this lovely paragraph:

> I do not think that a description of the earth, which commences, by telling a child that it is an oblate spheroid, moving round the sun in an elliptical orbit; and ends, without giving him the slightest hint towards understanding the ordnance map of his own county; or any suggestion as to the meaning of the phenomena offered by the brook which runs through his village, or the gravel pit whence the roads are mended; is calculated either to interest or to instruct. And the attempt to convey scientific conceptions, without the appeal to observation, which can alone give such conceptions firmness and

> reality, appears to me to be in direct antagonism to the fundamental principles of scientific education.

One could only wish that Huxley's larger views were more in sympathy with ours; but these words at least may illuminate some of what I had begun to say about the way that children begin to build relationships with the objects on the earth and in the heavens. I came across something else Huxley wrote which may be of use to us:

> Do not allow yourselves to be misled by the common notion that a hypothesis is untrustworthy simply because it is a hypothesis. It is often urged, in respect to some scientific conclusion, that, after all, it is only a hypothesis. But what more have we to guide us in nine tenths of the most important affairs of daily life than hypotheses, and often very ill-based ones?

Have you ever known a child who perhaps had a wrong understanding of something, because of their limited experience, but at the same time showed that they were putting their intelligence and imagination to work on the problem? Or perhaps you can think of other examples of the ways that we often simply follow our hypotheses.

Miss White: I'm thinking of scientists who go down a wrong track, but who learn something by the mistakes they make.

Miss Breckenridge: What about children who mishear things in stories, or words in songs? At least you know they've been paying attention, even if they don't get all the details right.

Miss Bruce: I think it's like the things our grandmothers told us to do or not to do, that for a long time were thought to be just "old wives' tales."

Miss Capehart: Right, like eating the…shall we say, not-as-fancy parts of animals. In the old days, people just handed down the idea that those things were good for you, or that there was some kind of luck or magic in it. Now people like Dr. Hopkins are discovering "accessory food factors" that keep us healthy.

Miss Glass: Sometimes the grandmothers were right all along, but sometimes not. I think the jury's still out on sitting on cement.

Miss Mason: I think we will end there, with this thought: when we consider that the setting up of relations, moral and intellectual, is our chief concern in life, and that the function of education is to put the child in the way of relations proper to him, and to offer the inspiring idea which commonly initiates a relation, we perceive that little examples like the ones you have shared may be of more importance than the passing of an examination.

Study 10: In Which Miss Mason Defends Herbart

Part One

Miss Mason: Today we will re-examine the work of Herbart, with the specific purpose of observing which fundamental ideas, long the property of the world, and which we have embraced in our own scheme of thought, appealed with equal force to so great and original a thinker.

I have indicated already what appears to me the root-defect of Herbartian educational philosophy—that it tends to eliminate personality, and therefore leads to curious futilities in teaching. But it needs to be seen how strong an educational force Herbart has been in Germany, especially as the successor of much older educators such as Comenius, Basedow, and Ratich.

Have you heard of Basedow? He was an eighteenth-century educator who brought nature study, physical education, and manual training into schools, and who argued against rote memorization and physical punishments. And Ratich? That name you will not hear much now, but he was an influence on Comenius. He believed that children should first study their mother tongue before learning other languages, and he also promoted inductive learning, especially in the study of nature. Consider that these were the educators, along with Pestalozzi and Froebel, who were most likely to have influenced Herbart.

But it is Herbart, and Herbart only, whose educational ideas are now followed in Germany, at least as much as is practical, since it has now been several decades since his death. We therefore have a unique opportunity to see Herbart's philosophy applied in what we may call its purest form, and to compare it to our own. And we are able to do so particularly because of this little volume, the *Outlines of Pedagogics* by Professor W. Rein of the University of Jena, which you may find in the library.

Now, first of all, we need to clarify some particular terminology. In some of your course papers, I have seen reference to Herbart, and the belief that a chief business of education, in *Herbart's* view, is to "develop the faculties." This is, however, not quite correct. Those ideas belong to the earlier reformers, notably Pestalozzi and Froebel, and of course Locke as well. What set Herbart apart from the rest was actually his *rejection* of the idea of faculties as something that could be neatly mapped out or packaged, the idea that certain school subjects were only to be used, for example, for developing one or the other faculty.

Now there was a certain pleasing neatness in the idea of separate faculties which was very attractive to the minds of educators in the past century. As teachers, we like to know what we have to do to attain a particular result, and this philosophy offered that. Why, develop the perceptive faculties here, with the conceptive there, the judgment in this lesson, the affections in the other, until you have covered the whole ground, giving each so-called faculty its due share of developmental exercise! That sheds much light on Pestalozzi's use of "object lessons." And that is also the theory by which the block work, and the games or "gifts" of the Froebelian Kindergarten were so carefully designed. But, say the followers of Herbart, we have changed all that. As train cars do not move alone, the mind moves *altogether* when it moves at all.

Now I am sympathetic to those who have been confused by this matter. I may have inadvertently misled you myself by a general reference to the German educationalists; and if so, I apologize. But this is something we need to see clearly, as it appears to be but a slight fundamental difference; but it is one upon the recognition of which education changes front. In Herbartian thought, the whole previous system of beautifully organized lessons, whose object is to develop this or that faculty, is called in question; there is no reason to continue such mental gymnastics if we no longer recognize particular "muscles" of the mind as needing to be developed. The aim of education must be something quite other, and, if the *aim* is other, the *methods* must be altered, for what is method but *a way to an end*?

So far we are entirely with Herbart. Where else do we find ourselves agreeing with him? In his recognition of the force of an *idea*, and especially of those ideas which are, as we phrase it, in the air at any given moment. He writes this:

> Both the circle of the family and that of social intercourse are subjected to forces that are active in the entire social body, and that penetrate the entire atmosphere of human life in invisible channels. No one knows whence these currents, these ideas arise; but they are there. They influence the moods, the aspirations, and the inclinations of humanity, and no one, however powerful, can withdraw himself from their effects; no sovereign's command makes its way into their depths. They are often born of a genius to be seized upon by the multitude that soon forgets their author; then the power of the thought that has thus become active in the masses again impels the individual to energetic resolutions: in this manner it is constantly describing a remarkable circle. Originating with those that are highly gifted, these thoughts permeate all society, reaching, in fact, not only its adult members, but also through these its youth, and appearing again in other highly gifted individuals in whom they will perhaps have been elevated to a definite form.
>
> Whether the power of these dominant ideas is greater in the individual, or in the body of individuals as a whole, is a matter of indifference here. Be that as it may, it cannot be denied that their effect upon the one is manifested in a reciprocal action upon the other, and that their influence upon the younger generation is indisputable.

We entirely agree that no one can escape the influence of this *Zeitgeist*, and that it is, in fact, one of the most powerful of the "supernatural" educational influences, and one which parents and all who have the training of children will do well to reckon with in the adjustment of their work. The list of those influences or "schoolmasters" includes Nature, family, "social intercourse," this *Zeitgeist*, the Church, and the State; but

Herbart considers, as do we, that by far the most valuable part of education is carried on in the *family*, because of the union of all the members, under a common parentage; because of the feeling of dependence upon a head; and because of the very intimate knowledge to be gained of the younger members. The members of the family look confidently to the head; and this sense of dependence favours, at the same time, the proper reception of that which is dearest to humankind, namely, the *religious* feeling. If the life of the family is permeated by a noble piety, a sincere religious faith take root in the hearts of the children. Faithful devotion to the guide of the youth also calls forth faithful devotion to Him who controls human destinies–a thought which Herbart expresses so beautifully with these words–"To the child, the family should be the symbol of the order in the world; from the parents one should derive, by idealization, the characteristics of the deity."

We will continue shortly with our detailed examination of Herbart's philosophy; but I want to illustrate the points already stated about "order in the world" reflecting the "characteristics of the deity." Miss Bruce, will you please pass these art prints out to the class? Take a few minutes to study the picture, and then I will add my comments.

Part Two

Miss Mason: Have any of you visited the Basilica of Santa Maria Novella in Florence? In the former chapter house of the convent there, we may see the Spanish Chapel, which was commissioned in the fourteenth century by a man named Buonamico Guidalotti, to be used as his funerary chapel. This picture at which you have been looking is part of the large fresco covering the walls and the vaulted ceiling. Who painted it? We have always thought that two artists named Taddeo Gaddi and Simone Memmi should get the credit for this work–so Mr. Ruskin has said in his useful book *Mornings in Florence*–but I have been told that Andrea da Firenze is the more likely artist.

The portion you are looking at is called *The Allegory of Christian Learning*, and it is found on the left wall. Here we have represented the descent of the Holy Ghost upon the Twelve Apostles; and directly under them, fully under the illuminating rays, are the noble figures of the seven liberal arts, which are Grammar, Rhetoric, Logic, Music, Astronomy, Geometry, and Arithmetic; and under these again the men who received and expressed, so far as the artist knew, the initial *idea* in each of these subjects: such men as Pythagoras, Zoroaster, and Euclid, whom *we* might call pagans, but whom the earlier Church recognized as divinely taught and illuminated.

Recall where we began this discussion—with Herbart's view of order in the world coming from one Head, that is, God. That is what I want you to understand here: that the medieval mind had that same understanding of God's Spirit illuminating all the different kinds of knowledge. Ruskin described it as "the teaching power of the Spirit of God, and the saving power of the Christ of God, in the world, according to the understanding of Florence in his time."

This idea of all education springing from and resting upon our relation to Almighty God is one which we have ever laboured to enforce. We take a very distinct stand upon this point. We do not merely give a *religious* education, because that would seem to imply the possibility of some *other* education, a secular education, for example. But we hold that all education is divine; that every good gift of knowledge and insight comes from above; that the Lord the Holy Spirit is the supreme educator of humankind; and that the culmination of all education (which may, at the same time, be reached by a little child) is that personal knowledge of and intimacy with God in which our being finds its fullest perfection.

Here are some final thoughts to consider, from *Mornings in Florence*:

> Here, then, you have pictorially represented, the system of manly education, supposed in old Florence to be that necessarily instituted in great earthly kingdoms or republics, animated by the Spirit shed down upon the world at Pentecost. How long do you think it will take you, or ought to take, to see such a picture? [If you visit Florence,] you have probably allowed half an hour for Santa Maria Novella; half an hour for San Lorenzo; an hour for the museum of sculpture at the Bargello; an hour for shopping; and then it will be lunch time, and you mustn't be late, because you are to leave by the afternoon train, and must positively be in Rome to-morrow morning.
>
> Well, of your half-hour for Santa Maria Novella,—after Ghirlandaio's choir, Orcagna's transept, and Cimabue's Madonna, and the painted windows, have been seen properly, there will remain, suppose, at the utmost, a quarter of an hour for the Spanish Chapel.
>
> That will give you two minutes and a half for each side, two for the ceiling, and three for studying Murray's [guidebook] or mine. Two minutes and a half you have got, then—(and I observed, during my five weeks' work in the chapel, that English visitors seldom gave so much)—to read this scheme given you...of human spiritual education. In order to understand the purport of it, in any the smallest degree, you must summon to your memory, in the course of these two minutes and a half, what you happen to be acquainted with of the doctrines and characters of Pythagoras, Zoroaster, Aristotle, Dionysius the Areopagite, St. Augustine, and the emperor Justinian, and having further observed the expressions and actions attributed by the painter to these personages, judge how far he has succeeded in reaching a true and worthy ideal of them, and how large or how subordinate a part in his general scheme of human learning he supposes their peculiar doctrines properly to occupy.
>
> ... and though indeed I came here from Lucca in three hours instead of a day, which it used to take, I do not think myself able, on that account, to see any picture in Florence in less time than it took formerly, or even obliged to hurry myself in any investigations connected with it.

If you want more detail on this, I recommend reading the chapter "The Vaulted Book," for yourselves. But please keep the copies of the picture; and you may take all the time you like to muse on it, since we are not rushing for the train. In fact, we may find ourselves referring back to it in future talks.

Part Three

Let us continue our reading of Herbart, as summarized by Dr. Rein. Here follows a passage which we do more than endorse, for it contains the very *raison d'être* of our society—the reason that we first formed the Parents' Union.

> The education of the children will always remain the holiest and highest of all family duties...The family principle is the point at which both the religious and educational life of a people centres, and about which it revolves. It is a force in comparison with which every sovereign's command appears powerless.

And I cannot take the time right now to do more than simply agree that, on that point, we have no argument with Herbart. As to the rest of Dr. Rein's book: after investigating the conditions of home training, which you can pursue further yourselves if you like, he proceeds to a discussion of schools (a) as they exist in Germany; and (b) as they exist in his own ideal, a discussion which should be most interesting to parents. Again, we cannot take more than that quick description right now, as, like Mr. Ruskin's tourists, we must portion out our time carefully, and there is one more item of special interest left us to discuss. That is *Teleology*: the theory of the purpose of education.

I would like you to get into groups of three, and discuss this question for exactly four minutes: what is the ultimate purpose of education?

Part Four

Miss Mason: Miss Laurio, how did your group answer this *teleological* question?

Miss Laurio: We thought that it would differ greatly depending on one's viewpoint. For instance, we ourselves liked the phrase "to prepare children for citizenship," but we thought that many others would say "to prepare them to know how to work."

Miss Mason: And Miss Capehart's group?

Miss Capehart: We have learned that education is the science of relations, and that a child is put into the world for the express purpose of forming ties of intimacy, joy, association, and knowledge with the living and moving things that are in it. So we focused on building relationships.

Miss Mason: As a matter of fact, few of us do know definitely what we propose to ourselves in the education of children. We do not know what it is possible to effect, and, as a man does not usually compass more than he aims at, the results of our education are inadequate and unsatisfactory...perhaps a bit like Ruskin's view that there was never enough time to fully appreciate the frescoes of Florence.

Let us hear the views of Herbart on some of the earlier educators, and the vast uncertainty which exists on this fundamental point.

> Shall the educator follow Rousseau and educate a man of nature in the midst of civilised men? In so doing... we should simply repeat from the beginning the entire series of evils that have already been surmounted. Or shall we turn to Locke and prepare the pupil for the world which is customarily in league with worldlings? We should then arrive at the standpoint of Basedow, and aim to educate the pupil so that he would become a truly useful member of human society. Of course we should always be harassed with the secret doubt as to whether this is ideal purpose after all, and whether we are not at times directly enjoined to place the pupil at variance with the usage and customary dealings of the world. If we reflect that an endless career is open to man for his improvement, we realise that only that education, whose aims are always the highest, can hope to reach the lofty goals that mark this career. Therefore an ideal aim must be present in the mind of the educator. Possibly he can obtain information and help from Pestalozzi, whose nature evinced such ideal tendencies. Pestalozzi wished the welfare of humankind to be sought in the "harmonious cultivation of *all* powers"...These phrases sound very attractive, but give little satisfaction.
>
> The purely *formal* aims of education will appeal as little to the educator: "Educate the pupil to independence"; or, "Educate the pupil to be his own educator"; or, "Educate the pupil so that 'it' will become better than 'its' educator." Such and similar attempts to fix the purpose of education are abundant in the history of pedagogy; but they do not bring us nearer the goal. In their formal character they do not say, for example, of what kind the independence shall be, what content it shall have, what aims it shall have in view, or in what directions its course shall lie. For the pupil that has become independent can use his freedom rightly for good just as well as misuse it for evil.

So we see that, oh yes, we do take a great risk as educators. Perhaps we may even educate too well, so that our students use what they have learned for evil instead of good! And is that fault then to be placed on the educator as much as the student? Sir John Adams, in his book *Herbartian Psychology*, has a most interesting passage on that question, but again, I can do no more right now than point you in that direction.

Well, what of Herbart's own theory, his view of the aims of education, after he has criticized all of these predecessors? Is he able to define an ultimate aim, and how much does it agree with our own? Herbart's own theory of education, so far as we may venture to formulate it, is strictly *ethical* as opposed to *intellectual.* Miss Bruce, how do you understand that?

Miss Bruce: He is saying that, strangely enough, educators should place only secondary importance on the development of the intellect, that character building is more important.

Miss Mason: Does it follow then that the intellect is to be depreciated, as, for instance, certain spiritual groups have believed? Yes, Miss Glass?

Miss Glass: According to Herbart, if we train character, then intellectual development largely takes care of itself. Oh, and I think he also said that the lessons designed for *intellectual* culture have high *ethical* value, whether they be "stimulating" or "disciplinary." So, for him, it all seems to come back to ethics.

Miss Mason: This is familiar ground to us: we too have taught, in season and out of season, that the *formation of character* is the aim of the educator. We do not downplay the work of the intellect by any means; but we place it in subjection to the higher values of character; and we also view it to be under the direction of the Holy Spirit.

Part Four

So far, we agree with the philosophy of Herbart; but–may we venture to say it?– we have arrived, through the study of Physiology, at the definiteness of aim which he desires but *does not reach.* I must speak of this main point of divergence only briefly today, but it is nonetheless of vital importance to us.

We must appeal, Herbart says, to Psychology. Now, you will recall *[Study 6]* that we have been looking for a system of educational Psychology that meets all the criteria we have set; and we crossed out several approaches because they failed to meet one or more of these points. Now Herbart also looks to Psychology itself for an answer to that question, "what is the aim of education?" But his conclusion is less than…conclusive. As Dr. Rein interprets him,

> Of course we cannot expect a concordant answer from all psychologists; and in view of the obscurity which still prevails in this sphere, the different views as to the nature of the human soul and the extraordinary difficulty with which the empirical method of investigation meets, an absolutely indubitable explanation can hardly be expected.

Herbart is admitting here that he does not know the answer; he does not believe that Psychology alone *can* provide an adequate answer to the "why" of education. Perhaps he believes that in this matter, he is labouring in the dark.

Well, with that much we do agree. This is doubtless true of Psychology alone.

However, of Psychology illuminated by Physiology we have another tale to tell. It is the study of that border-land betwixt mind and matter, the brain, which yields the richest results to the educator.

For the brain is the seat of *habit.*

The culture of habit is, to a certain extent, physical culture.

The discipline of habit is at least a third part of the great whole which we call education.

And here we feel that the *physical*, or physiological, science of today has placed us in advance of Herbart, the philosopher of fifty years ago. We hold with him entirely as to the importance of great formative ideas in the education of children, but we add to our ideas, habits; and we labour to form habits upon a *physical* basis.

We have stated that the aim of education is the formation of character. Character is the result not merely of the great *ideas* which are given to us, but of the *habits* which we labour to form upon those ideas. We recognize both of those principles, and the result is a wide range of possibilities in education, practical methods, and a definite aim. I have touched earlier on a few of those practical examples, but there is much more to say about them, and you have been supplied with readings on the various aspects of home training and classroom teaching. Your work in the Practising School will also give you the opportunity to apply those principles.

Let me close with this: we labour to produce a human being at his best physically, mentally, morally, and spiritually, with the enthusiasms of religion, of the good life, of nature, knowledge, art, and manual work; and we do *not* labour in the dark.

Study 11: A Serious Tea-Party

"It is my conviction that a system of education should have for its aim, not the mastery of certain 'subjects,' but the establishment of these relations in as many directions as circumstances will allow."

Part One

Miss Mason: I have reviewed the papers you submitted, outlining the ways that our work is unified and vitalized by a comprehensive theory of education and a sound basis of psychology. They were all quite well done, and I have added my comments. You may pick them up as you leave today.

We will begin with this much-used quotation: "Give me the child for the first seven years, and I will give you the man." Well, seven years is a start, but we would like to keep him till he is twelve or fourteen, if not a little longer. And you may do what you like with him afterwards.

[laughter]

Given this period for the establishing of relations, we may undertake to prepare for the world a man–or a woman–vital and vigorous, full of living interests, available and serviceable. I think we may warrant him, or her, even to pass the major examinations that seem to lie in everyone's way—because he or she will know how to put living interest into the dullest tasks.

Now, in a previous lecture we spoke at length about a child's relations with the world, particularly those that lead into the teaching of more formal sciences, through nature study and so forth. But we have not yet done with those relations. The second group of these are what I may call the *dynamic relations*: that is, *dynamic* as in the science of physics, those relationships involving motion. And we do want a child to experience many kinds of motion, particularly the sort he initiates him or herself. A child of normal physical ability must stand and walk and run and jump with ease and grace. He must skate and swim and ride and drive, dance and row and sail a boat. He should be able to make free with "Mother Earth," and to do whatever the principle of gravitation will allow. This is an elemental relationship for the lack of which nothing compensates.

Yes, Miss White? You have something to say?

Miss White: I'm sorry to sound petty, but many people don't live in climates where they can swim very much, or skate. Many children will never have the chance to sail a boat, or to ride horses; or they have no real inclination towards those things. On the other hand, there are parents who fill up the children's week with every sort of sport and activity, because it reassures them that they are providing everything possible for their children. Are we encouraging this anxiety to keep them constantly busy?

Miss Mason: First, to respond to your point about the child's own inclination or bent:

a great deal of wisdom and discrimination is needed here, especially regarding children who need to be pushed a little to play outdoors and try these different sorts of activities: we may take that as one of the situations where it would be more *arbitrary*, and less accepting of true *authority*, for the parent not to insist on at least a minimum of healthful energetic playtime, and outdoors whenever possible. There is no compensating later for a lack of such well-developed relations.

More generally, this is the *ideal* we are seeking. In the reading I will assign about the childhoods of Wordsworth and Ruskin, you will see that, certainly, no one situation is ideal; and where one person's early experience may be lacking in, as you say, the opportunity to ride horses (as you will hear in one of Ruskin's stories), it may be shored up by magnificent opportunities in some quite different area. Indeed, we cannot and should not try to create an absolutely perfect child-environment; as we have said, artificial perfection "stultifies" children. But we must do our best to provide what we can, wherever we live.

And as for the parents who rush their children from one lesson to another: I have said, and I will continue to say, that children require a great deal of time to develop these most important relationships, largely through play—and this is a sort of play in which adults must not interfere. So, no—although a class in gymnastics, for example, may offer much of value in teaching children to use their bodies, and will certainly give them good exercise, they also need time and space to learn and practice the sorts of movement that will come naturally. Who has not noticed that, if there is an old fallen log, children will invariably walk along it rather than beside it? Or that if there are stumps, they will jump from them? Or that if there is a ball or something else handy on the ground, they will kick it? Or that if there is enough of that wonderful plaything called snow, they will discover ways to slide and dig and stomp in it? Or that if there is a muddy puddle...well, you know the rest. And if children do not have the time to discover these things on their own, they will miss out greatly, not just in a sentimental sense, but in some vital connection, a relationship that should have been formed, which may or may not be able to be restored later on.

Now, we must speak of the third elemental relationship, which every child should be taught and encouraged to set up: that of *power over material*. Every child makes sand castles, mud-pies, paper boats...yes, Miss White, I am aware that not every child lives near the shore and can make sand castles every day, but still I am speaking of basic activities, that children seem to carry on wherever and whenever they live, with whatever materials come most readily to hand. And do children not have occasional holidays where they *do* encounter sand and water? My point here is that few children need to be *shown* how to do these simple things...they need only the material and the opportunity. And after those first relationships are established, a child should go on to work in clay, wood, brass, iron, leather, fabric, food-stuffs, furnishing materials...not all of them at once, of course, but as many as possible; and those things he perhaps cannot try for himself yet, he should also have the opportunity to watch older people doing. He should be able to make things with his hands, and should take *delight* in the making. Remember that we view this relationship as yet another connection with the earth, so we speak most particularly, really almost exclusively, of those materials that come in one way or other from the earth. Wool yarn, basketry materials, wood and metal provide, we may say, not a supernatural, but at least a *natural* connection with those things in the world around us.

And the fourth relationship children must establish is to the animal kingdom: a relation of intelligent comprehension as well as of kindness. Every child longs for intimacy with the creatures about him; and, as Coleridge wrote—

> He prayeth best, who loveth best
> All things both great and small;
> For the dear God who loveth us,
> He made and loveth all.

Part Two

Now we have described most of the non-human relationships, but what about the human ones? The relationships of love and service, of authority and obedience, of reverence and pity and neighbourly kindness; relationships to kin and friend and neighbour, to "cause" and country and kind, to the past and the present.

But they are not only developed through those persons directly around us. History, literature, archeology, art, languages, whether ancient or modern, travel and tales of travel; all of these are in one way or other the record or the expression of persons; and we who are persons are interested in all persons, for we are all one flesh, we are all of one spirit, and whatever any of us does or suffers is interesting to the rest. If we will approach them with living thought, living books, if we will only awaken in them the sense of personal relation, there are thousands of boys and girls to-day capable of becoming great leaders in government or diplomacy who can unite diverse groups of people. Or great archeologists who will make the past alive for us and make us aware in our souls of those who lived thousands of years ago. It rests with us to give the awakening idea and then to form the habit of thought and of life.

As an example of this aim, I have asked Miss Glass to present her notes of an oral lesson which she plans to give on the pictures of Fra Angelico. The students here are about sixteen years of age, so we will look at this with extra interest, remembering that our method here will not be identical to the way we would approach a lesson with young children, but that the need for *living ideas* remains the same. Miss Glass?

Miss Glass: We have half an hour for the class, and my objects are:

1. To show reproductions of some of Fra Angelico's pictures.
2. By means of them, to point out such distinguishing features as will enable my pupils to recognize Fra Angelico's work wherever they may see it.
3. To show in what degree his work holds a place in high art.

In this lesson, I plan to use these steps: Step One is to give a short sketch of the life of Fra Angelico. Step Two is to allow time for the students to look at the pictures provided, namely, various reproductions of "Christ in Glory," "Saints in Paradise,"

"Angels,' "Christ as Pilgrim, " "Annunciation," "Crucifixion," "Noli me tangere," "Descent from the Cross," and "Transfiguration."

Miss Mason: With a class of older students, we do not always have to confine ourselves to just one picture, as would be more typical for younger children.

Miss Glass: Step Three is to notice what strikes us most in Fra Angelico's work—the exquisite jewel-like finish; the pure open skies and unpretending clouds; the winding and abundant landscapes; the angels; the touches of white light; the delicacy and grace of form; the colouring; the peace. Of course I am hoping that the pupils will notice and comment on these things themselves.

And then for Step Four: If high art is to be seen "in the selection of a subject and its treatment, and the expression of the thoughts of the persons represented," as Ruskin says in *Modern Painters*, how far does Fra Angelico come up to this standard? Ruskin says that a painter's purpose is to combine the "perfect unison of expression with the full and natural exertion of his pictorial power." How does Fra Angelico illustrate this ideal of art? This will be illustrated by further reference to the pictures, and by reading some passages from *Modern Painters*.

Miss Mason: This is exactly the sort of idea that, we hope, leads to action, perhaps indirectly or in a different *mode*. Does not a writer wish to do a similar thing, for example? In any case, it offers ideas that may continue to be used as the students look at art in other places as well. Miss Glass, how will you end the lesson?

Miss Glass: I will allow my pupils time to look again at the pictures, asking them a few questions with the purpose of seeing if they have "caught" the main points. In a sense, this is their narration.

Miss Mason: I believe that, by this lesson and the others, you will have fulfilled your goal both of familiarizing the students with Fra Angelico's paintings, and also to show why his work does indeed "hold a place in fine art."

Miss Bruce: Miss Mason, how does that model of lesson planning translate to subjects that seem less capable of offering large human ideas, or of building relationships? Like a language lesson?

Miss Mason: There seems good reason to believe that the limit to human *intelligence* arises largely from the limit to human *interests,* that is, from the failure to establish personal relations on a wide scale with the persons who make up humanity,—relations of love, duty, responsibility, and, above all, of interest, living interest, with the near and the far-off, in time and in place. We hammer away for a dozen years at one or two languages, ancient or modern, and rarely know them very well at the end of that time, but directly they become to us the languages of persons whom we are aching to get at and can only do so through the medium of their own tongues, there seems no reason why many of us should not become multilingual.

Here is an example that one of the upper-class students submitted for a German grammar class of thirteen-year-olds [*Appendix B*]. The subject at hand is the construction of sentences, which, as the teacher notes, can seem very much complicated; yet with the help of a few simple rules it can be made much clearer. The question of technique here is whether we use a deductive or inductive method of teaching, whether we simply state the grammar rule and give examples, or whether the students try to work out the rule *from* examples. Using one method or the other is not a black-and-white issue for us, though we believe that, wherever possible, the inductive method helps the students to use their own powers of mind, with more success.

Note that students are frequently encouraged to translate the teacher's examples, to notice and reason out for themselves what is going on, and to put their own sentences on the blackboard *to show that they thoroughly understand the rule.*

Also note that this lesson has a clear structure and goals: to review what is known, to bring out just one or two new points, and then to recapitulate. Has it served the purpose of giving the students new power over language, of further opening the door to this specific language and the people who use it? I would say that it has, if only to demonstrate that the German language is not at all random, but that its word order follows specific rules. The teacher might suggest to the students that they look for examples in their own practice reading, whether of Scripture or some other sort of book or paper depending on their ability.

For those of you with little interest in German, this process can also be useful in planning a lesson in English grammar, in mathematics, or in science.

We will now take a short break. When the bell rings, please meet outside at the tea-table that is being set up in the garden. It is too nice a day to confine ourselves to this lecture-room, so we will take advantage of the sunshine.

Part Three (Around the Tea Table)

Miss Capehart: What do you think it would take to have a great educational revolution in this country?

Miss Glass: Imagine what lessons would be like if that were the case. History would become entrancing, literature, a magic mirror for the discovery of other minds.

Mr. Miller (a visitor whose business it is to read manuscripts for a publishing firm): We would have to see ourselves, and the children, as persons whose great business it is to get in touch with other persons of all sorts and conditions, of all countries and climes, of all times, past and present.

Miss Laurio: Well, there, you have put both the first and second PNEU principles into one sentence! Admirable.

Miss Breckenridge: We should tend to become more responsive and wise, humble and reverent, recognizing the duties and the joys of the full human life.

Miss White: Even the study of sociology would be a duty and a delight—says one who is not fond of sociology class.

Miss Laurio: Did you ever turn in that overdue paper?

Miss White: I'm working on it.

Miss Glass: I think sociology *is* important. It implies a practical relation with other people which children should begin to get, and it is a kind of knowledge they seem very ready for. The carpenter, the gardener, the baker, the candlestick maker, are all delightful persons in a child's eyes; and it is surprising how much a child visiting the seaside will get to know about boats and sails and fishermen's lives. In later years when he hears about workers on strike, or he has to consider other causes and questions of justice, he will think of those people, and their crafts and trades, behind the impersonal words in the news stories.

Miss Capehart: Of course that is one place where literature helps us, since we cannot all meet bakers and candlestick makers.

Miss Mason: We cannot, of course, overtake such a programme of work, but we can keep it in view; and, I suppose, every life is moulded upon its ideal. We talk of lost ideals, but perhaps they are not lost, only changed; when our ideal for ourselves and for our children becomes limited to *prosperity* and *comfort*, we get these, very likely, for ourselves and for them; but we get no more.

Let us consider the ideal of "duty." If we believe that a person is no more than a "state of consciousness" *[Study 6]*, well then, we cannot be expected to take up moral responsibilities, except such as appeal to us at the moment. Duty, in the sense of relations imposed by authority and *due* to our fellows, does not fall within the scope of present-day psychology. If we do not recognize outside authority *[Study 1]*, and if we do not have responsibility to others, then duty does not exist.

In the Church of England catechism, when children are taught to say the Ten Commandments, they follow them with these questions:

> *Question.* What dost thou chiefly learn by these Commandments?
> *Answer.* I learn two things; my duty towards God, and my duty towards my Neighbour.
> *Question.* What is thy duty towards God?
> *Answer.* My duty towards God, is to believe in him, to fear him, and to love him with all my heart, with all my mind, with all my soul, and with all my strength; to worship him, to give him thanks, to put my whole trust in him, to call upon him, to honour his holy Name

> and his Word, and to serve him truly all the days of my life.
> *Question.* What is thy duty towards thy Neighbour?
> *Answer.* My duty towards my Neighbour, is to love him as myself, and to do to all men, as I would they should do unto me: To love, honour, and succour my father and mother: To honour and obey the civil authority: To submit myself to all my governors, teachers, spiritual pastors and masters: To order myself lowly and reverently to all my betters: To hurt nobody by word or deed: To be true and just in all my dealings: To bear no malice nor hatred in my heart: To keep my hands from picking and stealing, and my tongue from evil speaking, lying, and slandering: To keep my body in temperance, soberness, and chastity: Not to covet nor desire other men's goods; but to learn and labour truly to get mine own living, and to do my duty in that state of life unto which it shall please God to call me.

Mr. Miller: I am more familiar with Luther's Small Catechism, which follows each commandment with the question "What does this mean?" For instance, the commandment "Thou shalt honour thy father and thy mother" is followed with "What does this mean? We should fear and love God that we may not despise nor anger our parents and masters, but give them honour, serve, obey, and hold them in love and esteem." And "Thou shalt not kill," which most children would think does not apply much to them, is followed by the explanation that "We should fear and love God that we may not hurt nor harm our neighbor in his body, but help and befriend him in every bodily need." Suddenly it becomes more pertinent.

Miss Mason: With the Ten Commandments (and such catechisms) as a basis, children used to get a fairly thorough ethical teaching from the Bible. They knew the mandates "Love the brethren," "Fear God," "Honour the King," "Honour all men," "Study to be quiet." They knew that thoughts of hatred and contempt were of the nature of murder. They knew what King Solomon said of the virtuous woman, of the sluggard, of the fool. Their knowledge was not confined to precepts; from history, sacred and profane, they were able to illustrate every text. We in England have not the wealth of moral teaching carved in wood and stone which some neighbouring countries rejoice in; but our teaching, until the present generation, has been systematic and thorough.

Miss Capehart: Do you not see it as such now?

Miss Mason: I will ask that myself of Mr. Miller. What is your experience with this in the publishing field, and in the books that parents and teachers ask for these days?

Mr. Miller: Many parents say that they eschew for the children (and often wisely!) all stories with a moral; their books must be amusing, and they ask little more. Others require that the books must be literary, and then, perhaps, a little instructive. But they do not look for a "moral impulse" fitly given. It is not that they give no ethical teaching, but their teaching is casual. If teachers or parents happen on a story of heroism or self-denial, they seem glad to point the moral. But children rarely get now a distinct ethical system resting on the broad basis of the brotherhood of man.

Miss Mason: We may disdain it as merely parroting if a child recites "My duty towards my Neighbour, is to love him as myself" and "to do to all men, as I would they should do unto me"; but the fact is that most ten-year-old children cannot even recite these words today, much less carry them out.

Mr. Miller: A great many fine things are said to-day about the brotherhood of man and the solidarity of the race, but I think we shall look in vain in modern writings for a sentence which goes to the root of the matter as does this authoritative code of duty.

Miss Mason: If the whole of education consists in the establishment of relations, then the relations with our fellow-beings must be of the first importance, do you not agree?

Mr. Miller: Yes, barring the relationship with our heavenly Father.

Miss Mason: Then all associations formed upon any basis except that of "my duty towards my neighbour,"–as upon *sympathy* in art or literature, for example,–are apt to degenerate into sentimental bonds; and the power of original thought appears curiously to depart with that of moral insight. We must feel that sense of duty and responsibility for each other's well-being—or we will find ourselves only fair-weather friends.

Miss Breckenridge: Is there some other way to get a scheme of ethical teaching for our children, if we choose to forego the Ten Commandments and the old-fashioned ways of explaining them?

Miss Mason: There are a thousand *supplementary* ways of giving such teaching; but these are apt to be casual and little binding if they do not rest upon the solid foundation of *duty* imposed upon us by God (so recognizing His authority), and *due* to each other, whether we will or no. This moral relation of person to person underlies all other relations. We owe it to the past to use its gains worthily and to advance from the point at which it left off. We owe it to the future to prepare a generation better than ourselves. We owe it to the present to *live*, to live with all expansion of heart and soul, all reaching out of our personality towards those relations appointed for us. We owe knowledge to the ignorant, comfort to the distressed, healing to the sick, reverence, courtesy and kindness to all men, especially to those with whom we are connected by ties of family or neighbourhood; and the sense of these dues does not come by nature.

Miss Glass: What of children who grow up in "good homes," but who are untrained in their moral relations?

Miss Mason: That is a sad state of neglect. Any young person should be made familiar with such a working system of psychology or philosophy, whichever one likes to call it, as shall help him to conduct his relations with himself and with other people. Even the ancients sent their children to school for instruction in philosophy. And notice that I used the phrase "with himself." Modern scientists have added a great deal to the sum of available knowledge which should bear on the conduct of those relations of oneself with *oneself* which are implied in terms such as self-management, self-control, self-respect, self-love, self-help, self-abnegation, and so on. This knowledge is the more important because our *power* to conduct our relations with other people depends upon our *power* of conducting our relations with ourselves *[Study 26]*.

Mr. Miller: And if we learn something from our own person about such a key to human nature, and in proportion as we are able to use that key, we shall become not more dictatorial, but more tolerant, gentle, helpful, wise and reverent. If we have no understanding of those springs of conduct common to us all, if we are not able to conduct ourselves well, then we will not be able to expect anything much of those who work for us or serve us, or who we are given responsibility for as parents. Or, as teachers, you will not expect much "evolution of the person" from your students, and the results will be in proportion.

Miss White: So we do not then simply give up a child to be selfish, or greedy, or lazy. A child who has been "cured" of some such blemish will not be slow to believe when he grows up in the possibility of reform for others, and in the use of simple, practical means. And if we have seen these methods create improvement in our own lives, we know that they will work for others as well.

Miss Mason: I think we may really give a little credit to the PNEU for an advance in this direction. Most people associated with us know something of the treatment of sensations, the direction of the will, the treatment of temper, the psychology of attention, the desires and affections which are the springs of conduct, and other practical matters concerned with the management of one's life. We hear of people who use that fine old nursery plan, "change your thoughts," with method and success in the case of adults as well. We feel as if we had a tool in our hands and knew how to set to work. The principle, anyhow, we perceive to be right; and, if we blunder in its application, we try again, whether for ourselves or for our children.

Miss Bruce: Do you have a particular plan in this area for young people?

Miss Mason: The value of self-managed clubs and committees, debating societies, etc., is becoming more and more fully recognized. Organizing capacity, business habits, and some power of public speaking, should be a part of our fitness as citizens. But to secure the power of speaking, I think it would be well if the habit of oral narration were more encouraged in schools, in place of written composition. On the whole, it is more useful to be able to speak than to write, and the man or woman who is able to do the former can generally do the latter.

Miss Glass: Miss Mason, you spoke earlier of our "duty towards God." Would you have any more to say about that now?

Miss Mason: How many children are to-day taught to say at their mother's knee, to learn from day to day and from hour to hour, in all its fulness of meaning, those words from the catechism— "My duty towards God, is to believe in him, to fear him, and to love him with all my heart, with all my mind, with all my soul, and with all my strength; to worship him, to give him thanks, to put my whole trust in him, to call upon him, to honour his holy Name and his Word, and to serve him truly all the days of my life?" Whether children are taught their duty towards God in these or other words matters little; but I fear that many children grow up untaught in these matters. The idea of *duty* is not wrought into the very texture of their souls; and *duty* to Him who is invisible, which should be the very foundation of life, is least taught of all. I do not say that children are allowed to grow up without religious sentiments and religious emotions, and that they do not say quaint and surprising things, showing that they have an insight of their own into the higher life. But duty and sentiment are two different things. Sentiment is optional; and young people grow up to think that they *may* believe in God, *may* fear God, *may* love God in a measure—but that they *must* do these things, that there is no choice at all about the love and service of God, that it is their duty, that which they *owe*, to love Him "with all their heart, with all their mind, with all their soul, with all their strength," these things are seldom taught and understood as they should be.

Even where our sentiment is warm, our religious notions are lax; and children, the children of good, religious parents, who have not been given that sense of "ought," grow up without that intimate, ever-open, ever-cordial, ever-corresponding relation with Almighty God, which is the very fulfilment of life. One cannot exist without the other.

Miss Laurio, would you close our discussion by reading these lines I have marked from Robert Browning?

Miss Laurio:

> I want,—am made for, —and must have a God,
> Ere I can be aught, do aught; —no mere Name
> Want, —but the True Thing, with what proves its truth,
> To wit, a relation from that Thing to me,
> Touching from head to foot—which Touch I feel,
> And with it take the rest, this Life of ours!

Notes for a New Era

On Sociology

In *Study 11*, Miss Glass says, "I think sociology *is* important…" Literary critic Alan Jacobs agrees:

> [Sociologists of the early 20th century] differentiated themselves from earlier humanistic thought in some interesting and useful ways.
>
> One of the key such differentiations is the emphasis, in early sociology and anthropology, on the continuities of human experience. That is, though these thinkers were certainly highly aware of the dramatically different social practices that could be found in the cultures of the world, and researched those varying practices with great care and thoroughness, they nevertheless believed that there were certain permanent human impulses that make their way into every culture.
>
> The most important conclusion to be drawn from that insight is that our belief in ourselves as modern persons, or rational persons, different from the primitives who preceded us and who still might persist in strange corners of the world, is an illusion. We are driven by the same needs as all others humans past and present. (Jacobs, 2022a)

What educational practices do you find most useful in promoting "the solidarity of the race?"

On the Disunity of Unit Studies

Unit studies have long been popular with homeschoolers, for various reasons: they provide opportunity for older and younger children to work together, especially when there is a desire to get away from grade-leveled material; they can involve both books and hands-on activities, and may (if well done) encourage research skills; and they seem to provide the natural framework of a specific topic, although (as Miss Breckenridge points out in *Study 7*) some topics could go on indefinitely. The culminating projects of unit studies are often challenging and creative. For those who are used to textbook/workbook methods, unit studies may feel like a breath of fresh air.

However, Miss Mason says, "If one is to find the principles of unity and continuity in the ideas presented to the soul, this is all good and well. But if, as we believe, these principles must *emanate* from the soul, or *person*, him or herself, this tempting 'unity' [offered by unit study plans] may result in the collection of a mass of scattered and unassimilated information." In other words: making too many connections *for* the students results in the reverse effect: what they do not "scratch out" for themselves may end up merely scattered to the side. This may not be a popular point of view, but if we believe that students must be allowed to form their own relationships, it does make sense.

Have you used some form of unit studies in your teaching? What were the advantages or disadvantages? What middle ground is offered here instead?

Other Thoughts

If the root-defect of Herbart's educational philosophy is that it tends to eliminate personality, how does that lead to "curious futilities" in teaching? Consider that Herbart had not only become the dominant educational force in Germany by the twentieth century, as Miss Mason said, but also that he is *still* a major influence on North American education decades later. Can you see a correlation between, for example, the school education you received yourself, and the philosophy of Herbart?

Mary Pride's book *Schoolproof* (1994) was not so much an indictment of the public school system as it was a warning to home educators not to imitate the "clutter" typical of that system. If you are currently teaching one, two, or more students, in any situation, do you find yourself struggling to decrease "clutter" and "futilities," or even to discern what those are? Here is one suggestion: begin by putting the focus on "personality," and see if that makes the choices clearer. Part of the "personality" that Miss Mason saw lacking in Herbart's educational philosophy had to do with "add[ing] to our ideas, habits; and we labour to form habits upon a *physical* basis." She gave Herbart the benefit of the doubt on this, saying that he did not have the advantage of recent advances in neurological science; but in any case, she believed that habit was one of the next important steps in education. When you put the words "habit" and "personality" together, does it feel like a contradiction? Make a Venn diagram of the two, or simply list the characteristics of each one and try to see why Miss Mason considered "habit" to be foundational to an education grounded in "personality."

Another quote: "Such a system *may* turn out good mathematicians and clear-headed scientists; but what place is there in it for the higher forces of humanity, aspiration, speculation, devotion?" Out of these words, are there any that you find difficult to define? "Speculation" might cause some trouble, as it doesn't seem that Miss Mason was referring to either the stock market or simply guessing at answers to a question. However, it can also carry the meaning of contemplation or consideration on important matters, as in these lines by Wordsworth:

> Ye mountains! thine, O Nature! Thou hast fed
>
> My lofty speculations; and in thee,
>
> For this uneasy heart of ours I find
>
> A never-failing principle of joy,
>
> And purest passion.

Part Three: Surviving One's Childhood (In Which the Student Teachers Dissect Wordsworth and Ruskin)

A thoughtful writer has done us good service by carefully tracing the method of our Lord's education of the Twelve. "Our Lord," says this author, "reverenced whatever the learner had in him of his own, and was tender in fostering this native growth. . .Men, in His eyes, were not mere clay in the hands of the potter, matter to be moulded to shape. They were organic beings, each growing from within, with a life of his own—a personal life which was exceedingly precious in His and His Father's eyes—and He would foster this growth so that it might take after the highest type." (*Pastor Pastorum, or The Schooling of the Apostles by Our Lord*, by Rev. Henry Latham; quoted in *School Education*, p. 183.)

Study 12: Educated by Our Intimacies

"Most thinking people are in earnest about the bringing up of children; but we are in danger of taking too much upon us, and of not recognizing the limitations which confine us to the outworks of personality." "Outworks," in military terms, means the section of the defense that is ahead of, or outside of, the main part. To use a more biological metaphor, a cell membrane, of which we are forbidden to touch the inner parts.

However, that is more than sufficient for our purposes! Read on to find out how to teach and train while keeping to the limit of "three instruments."

Note on the quotations used in these studies: the lines from Wordsworth, unless otherwise noted, are from his long poem The Prelude, *which served as his autobiography in verse form. The Ruskin references are from his autobiography* Praeterita.

Prologue

Miss Mason: We know well that "Education is an atmosphere, a discipline, a life." In other words, parents and teachers should know how to make sensible use of a child's **circumstances** (*atmosphere*) to forward his sound education; should train him in the *discipline* of the **habits** of the good life; and should *nourish his life* with **ideas**, the food upon which personality waxes strong. These three we believe to be the *only* instruments of which we may make lawful use in the upbringing of children; and any short cut we take by trading on their sensibilities, emotions, desires, or passions, will bring us and our children to grief.

The reason is plain; habits, ideas, and circumstances are external, and we may all help each other to get the best that is to be had of these; but we may not meddle directly with the personality of child or man. We may not work upon his vanity, his fears, his love, his emulation, or anything that is his by right, anything that goes to make him a person.

As our Prospectus says *[Study 19]*,

> A child should be brought up to have relations of force with earth and water, should run and ride, swim and skate, lift and carry; should know texture, and work in material; should know by name, and where and how they live at any rate, the things of the earth about him, its birds and beasts and creeping things, its herbs and trees; should be in touch with the literature, art and thought of the past and the present.

All children should have dear and intimate relations with persons, through present interaction, or through tale or poem, picture or statue; through flint arrow-head or modern motor-car: beast and bird, herb and tree, with all these they must have familiar acquaintance. Other peoples and their languages must not be strange to them. Above all they should find that most intimate and highest of all Relationships—the fulfilment of their being.

Does that sound like a bewildering programme?

Not at all, because, in all these and more directions, children have affinities; and a human being does not fill his place in the universe without putting out tendrils of attachment in the directions proper to him. We must get rid of the notion that to learn the "three R's" or the Latin grammar well, a child should learn these and nothing else. It is as true for children as for ourselves that, the wider the range of interests, the more intelligent is the apprehension of each.

We do *not* talk about developing the child's faculties, training his moral nature, guiding his religious feelings, educating him with a view to his social standing or his future calling. *[Editor's note: Perhaps those should be considered the inner, untouchable parts of the cell.]* We take the child for granted, or rather, we take him as we find him—a person with an enormous number of healthy affinities, embryo attachments; and we think it is our chief business to give him a chance to make the largest possible number of these attachments valid.

But with all the errors that well-meaning parents and teachers make, with all the limitations and circumstances unique to any one childhood, how is it that many of us still manage to discover enough of our "personhood," and its attached "affinities," to carry us into a successful state of adulthood?

We do not offer this as an excuse to parents and teachers who might therefore shirk their responsibility, and certainly not so that they might hope to turn out a Poet Laureate! As St. Paul said, "What shall we say then? Shall we continue in sin, that grace may abound? (Romans 6:1)" We may not leave off the attempt to form good *habits* with tact and care, to suggest fruitful *ideas* (without too much insistence), and to make wise use of *circumstances*. The laws of habit are, we know, laws of God, and the forming of good and the hindering of evil habits are among the primary duties of a parent. But it is just as well to be reminded that *habits*, whether helpful or hindering, only come into play occasionally; while a great deal of spontaneous *living* is always going on towards which we can do no more than drop in vital ideas as opportunity occurs.

But indeed, I do not think we make enough use of two such priceless boons to parents and teachers as the educational autobiographies we possess of two great philosophers, William Wordsworth and John Ruskin. As part of your work, I have asked you to examine them each, looking particularly for examples of the relationships that they were able to form during childhood, including Dynamic Relations *[Study 11]*, Power Over Material *[Study 11]*, and *Historic Sense*. Today we will hear your reports from this assignment, and I may add in some comments as we go on.

Miss Breckenridge, will you begin with the early life of Wordsworth?

Part One: William Wordsworth

Miss Breckenridge: Wordsworth. Just think of it! A poet whose name evokes what he does, in that he takes words and makes them worthy. Wordsworth means the Lake District, a sleep and a forgetting, first-born affinities, the child is father of the man, a violet in a mossy stone, and always, a host of golden daffodils. Wordsworth's poetry includes approachable nature, recognizable emotions, and a picture of the relationship between the two. And sometimes he does it all "within the sonnet's scanty ground."

William Wordsworth was born in Cockermouth, England, in 1770, right here in the Lake District. He was the second of five children; his sister Dorothy, a poet in her own right, was born just a year after William and they were close all their lives. Their father, whose job took him away from the family for long stretches of time, provided his children with a home that included a library and a situation beside the Derwent River. So William grew up with access to great books and a rural paradise, and his poetry reflected that.

These lines from *The Prelude* describe the difficulty of trying to remember where or when some of one's first ideas appeared, but how one experience might nevertheless have been the spark of something important later on.

> But who shall parcel out
> His intellect by geometric rules,
> Split like a province into round and square?
> Who knows the individual hour in which
> His habits were first sown, even as a seed?
> Who that shall point as with a wand and say
> 'This portion of the river of my mind
> Came from yon fountain'?

Miss Mason: Thank you, Miss Breckenridge, that gives us a good beginning. Miss White, will you share your findings on Wordsworth?

Miss White: Miss Mason, I found something you wrote which says– may I read this?–

> We temper the wind too much to the lambs; pain and sin, want and suffering, disease and death—we shield them from the knowledge of these at all hazards. I do not say that we should wantonly expose the tender souls to distress, but that we should recognize that life has a ministry for them also; and that Nature provides them with a subtle screen, like that of its odour to a violet, from damaging shocks.

Some of us will not even let children read fairy tales because these bring the ugly facts of life too suddenly before them. I think it is natural for us to want to protect our children from anything that might hurt them, but that can also keep them from learning to deal with life's complications.

Consider Wordsworth's experience on this point. He tells us how, no sooner had he gone to school at Hawkshead, than a corpse was recovered from Esthwaite Lake; it is a ghastly tale, but full of comfort as showing how children are somewhat protected from shock.

> ...yet no soul-debasing fear,
> Young as I was, a child not nine years old,
> Possessed me, for my inner eye had seen
> Such sights before, among the shining streams
> Of fairyland, the forests of romance:
> Their spirit hallowed the sad spectacle

With decoration of ideal grace;
A dignity, a smoothness, like the works
Of Grecian art, and purest poesy.

Miss Mason: It is comforting to know, on the evidence of a child, that a terrible scene was separated from him by an atmosphere of poetry—a curtain woven of fairy lore by his etherealizing imagination. But we may run no needless risks, and must keep a quiet, matter-of-fact tone in speaking of fire, shipwreck, or any terror. There are children to whom the thought of Joseph in the pit [Genesis 37] is a nightmare; and many of us adults who are unable to endure a ghastly tale in newspaper or novel. All I would urge is a *natural* treatment of children, and that they be allowed their fair share of life, such as it is; prudence and not panic should rule our conduct towards them.

Miss Bruce, have you an example to put forward?

Miss Bruce: An infant comes with many "feelers," as we might call them…and he wants to find the right things to attach them to. As Wordsworth says of himself,

...the Babe,
Nursed in his Mother's arms...
No outcast he, bewildered and depressed:
Along his infant veins are interfused
The gravitation and the filial bond
Of nature that connects him with the world.

A young child attaches his being to mother, father, sister, brother, his "nanna and poppa," the man in the street whom he calls "da-da." The cat and dog, spider and fly; earth, air, fire, and water attract him perilously; his eyes covet light and colour, his ears sound, his limbs movement; everything concerns him, and out of everything he gets—

...that calm delight
Which, if I err not, surely must belong
To those first-born affinities that fit
Our new existence to existing things,
And, in our dawn of being, constitute
The bond of union between life and joy.

He gets also, when left to himself, the real knowledge about each thing which establishes his relation with that particular thing.

Miss Mason: Later, we step in to educate him. In proportion to the range of living relationships we put in his way, will he have wide and vital interests, fulness of joy in living. In proportion as he is made aware of the laws which rule every relationship, will his life be dutiful and serviceable: as he learns that no relation with persons or with things, animate or inanimate, can be maintained without strenuous effort, will he learn the laws of work and the joys of work. And again, what is education after all?

Everyone: "Education is the Science of Relations."

Part Two: John Ruskin

Miss Mason: I said earlier that "in proportion to the range of living relationships *we put* in a child's way, will he have wide and vital interests, fulness of joy in living." Our deadly error, however, is to suppose that we are the child's "showman to the universe"; and, not only so, but that there is no community, or relation, at all between child and universe unless such as *we* choose to set up. "We are the people!" we say; and if we choose that a village child's education should be confined to the "three R's," why, what right has he to ask for more? If he grows up and *life* means for him his Saturday night in the ale-house, surely that is not our fault!

And if more privileged children go through private schools and good colleges, and still come out without quickening interests, without links to the things that are worthwhile, we are not sure that it is our fault either. We resent that the college athletes should be called "flannelled fools at the wicket" or "muddied oafs at the goals," as Mr. Kipling wrote, because we know them to be fine fellows. So they are, splendid stuff which has not yet arrived at the making!

But is that not sad for them?

Hamlet said, "Every man hath business and desire," and doubtless that was true in the "spacious times of great Elizabeth" [Tennyson, *A Dream of Fair Women*]. But for us, we have business, but have we *desire*? Are there many keen *interests* soliciting us outside of our necessary work? Perhaps not, or we should be less enslaved by the vapid joys of Ping-Pong, card games, and the like. If you ask a young person what he or she likes to do, those are the replies you will often get—recent fads, popular pastimes, current sports. But the fact is that *interests* are not to be taken up on the spur of the moment; they spring out of affinities we have found and laid hold of.

Still the question remains, how to set about it. We will now hear something of the boyhood of John Ruskin from Miss Glass.

Miss Glass: John Ruskin, who lived from 1819 to 1900, was a writer, painter, social critic and philosopher; he was an expert on many subjects, and inspired many other writers and artists. Here we are most familiar with his fairy tale *The King of the Golden River*, his lectures *Ethics of the Dust*, and his books on travel and art, as well as his autobiography, *Praeterita*, which means "the past."

It is of particular interest to us that Ruskin was involved during the 1860's with a progressive school for girls at Winnington Hall in Cheshire, and that he encouraged the girls in their pursuits of sports, handicrafts, music, and dancing. He was also a mentor and benefactor to other women's colleges. He is known to have had a gentle demeanour, but has also been called "charismatic." When looking at the early influences on his character, his home life and so on, however, we recognize the fact that he was not always a happy man, and that some aspects of his adult life were indeed very difficult.

In 1839, Ruskin was honoured with the Newdigate Prize for poetry, given to undergraduate students at Oxford. (Arthur Hugh Clough, the editor of our Dryden

Plutarch, came in second). He met William Wordsworth, who was receiving an honourary doctorate in Civil Law, at the ceremony.

Miss Mason: Most interesting! What have you found out about his affinities, habits, character formation and the rest?

Miss Glass: You have said that a child should have Dynamic Relations with earth and water: that he or she must run and leap and dance, ride and swim and so forth. But this is how *not* to do it, as Ruskin recalls:

> My father spared time from his business hours, once or twice a week, to take me to a four-square, sky-lighted, saw-dust floored prison of a riding school in Moorfields, the smell of which, as we turned in at the gate of it, was a terror and horror and abomination to me: and there I was put on big horses that jumped and reared, and circled, and sidled, and fell off them regularly whenever they did any of these things; and was a disgrace to my family, and a burning shame and misery to myself, till at last the riding school was given up on my spraining my right hand fore-finger (it has never come straight again since); and a well-broken Shetland pony bought for me, and the two of us led about the Norwood roads by a riding master with a leading string.
>
> I used to do pretty well as long as we went straight, and then get thinking of something and fall off as we turned a corner. I might have got some inkling of a seat in heaven's good time, if no fuss had been made about me, nor inquiries instituted whether I had been off or on; but as my mother the moment I got home made searching scrutiny into the day's disgraces, I merely got more nervous and helpless after every tumble; and this branch of my education was at last abandoned, my parents consoling themselves as best they might, in the conclusion that my not being able to learn to ride was the sign of my being a singular genius.

Miss Mason: Ruskin was a child of the wealthy middle class who think, not wisely but too much, about the bringing up of their children, who choke a good deal of life with care and coddling, and are apt to be persuaded that their children want no outlets but such as it occurs to them to provide. With all his chivalrous loyalty to his parents, Ruskin has left here a grave indictment, not of them, but of the limitations of his condition, class, and lifestyle. One hears the cry of the child, like that of Laurence Sterne's caged starling–"I can't get out, I can't get out"–repeated from page to page. Suburban life is a necessity, but it is also a misfortune, because, in a rich suburb, people live too much with their own sort, and are cut off from both the small and the great.

You will say, whatever were the faults of his education, *Ruskin* emerged from it, and we look for no more, in the same way that great musicians and inventors and reformers have come out of poor beginnings. But it is not for us to say how much greater an apostle among men even Ruskin would have become, had he been allowed his right of free living as a child. And it may be, on the other hand, safe to admit that not every child, born and bred in a villa, will certainly be another Ruskin!

Miss Glass, have you more to add?

Miss Glass: We cannot follow Mr. Ruskin further in the setting up of "the dynamic relations proper to him," because his parents forbade, and nothing happened. His mother, he says, "never allowed me to go to the edge of a pond or be in the same field with a pony." But he notes "with thankfulness the good I got out of the tadpole-haunted ditch in Croxted Lane." Camberwell Green had a pond, and, he says, "it was one of the most valued privileges of my early life to be permitted by my nurse to contemplate this judicial pond with awe from the other side of the way."

Miss Mason: Indeed, a somewhat bittersweet choice of words there, for those of us who would prefer our children to put rubber boots on and explore the judicial pond themselves. Have you any questions regarding, particularly, Ruskin's comments on his childhood? We will be able to compare it more closely with that of Wordsworth in the next session.

Miss Capehart: Yes, to be frank, I find his complaining irritating. Certainly Ruskin's childhood had its limitations, but he certainly was quite privileged compared to many other children, both in his time and now. I don't feel especially sorry for the "poor" children of the wealthy: their parents can afford to do things like send them to lovely summer camps or take them on holidays where they can really sail and ride and all the rest of it, and buy them books and art supplies and construction toys. I'm more concerned with children who are actually abused or hungry or exposed to dangers.

Miss Laurio: Is it possible that we may be wasting our time trying to convince the wealthier class of parents that they could be living more creative lives themselves, and raising happier, more connected children? Some of us are drawn to "settlement work" in the cities, where the need seems to be greater but where small improvements can make big differences.

Miss Mason: I do not say that you are wrong, only that, as we said before, even the "flannelled fools" are "splendid stuff which has not yet arrived at the making." That is, they are the same "stuff" as you and I are made of, with the same desires, the same need to discover the things for which we are all created, and for which we have the same affinities.

And let me say a word as to the "advantages" which living in a large city offers in the way of masters and special classes. I think it is most often the still pool which the angel comes down to trouble (John 5:4); and a steady unruffled course of work without so-called advantages lends itself best to that "troubling" of the angel—the striking upon us of what Coleridge calls the "Captain Idea," which initiates a tie of affinity.

We will continue examining these questions when next we meet.

Study 13: Childhood Joys and Disappointments

Part One

Miss Mason: We earlier heard something of Ruskin's frustration over not being allowed "genuine" experiences. However, Wordsworth's bringing-up was more rough-and-tumble than that of Ruskin. Miss Laurio, can you elaborate?

Miss Laurio: When Wordsworth was nine, he was sent to the Grammar School in the little village of Hawkshead, and lodged with Dame Tyson in the cottage many of us know. He found most things, at home and abroad, congenial to his soul. He had no lessons in riding and skating, hockey and tennis; but no doubt the other boys made it plain to the little chap that he must do as they did or be thought a fool. But then he went to school a hardy youngster; his mother had let her little boy *live*:—

> Oh, many a time have I, a five years' child,
> In a small mill-race severed from his stream,
> Made one long bathing of a summer's day;
> Basked in the sun, and plunged, and basked again.

Of his childhood, he says:—

> Fair seed-time had my soul, and I grew up
> Fostered alike by beauty and by fear.

Before his tenth birthday, he was transplanted to that "beloved Vale" of which he says:—

> ...there were we let loose
> For sports of wider range.

It sounds like there was very little that those Hawkshead boys did not do! He tells us of times,—

> ...when I have hung
> Above the raven's nest, by knots of grass
> And half-inch fissures in the slippery rock
> But ill-sustained, and almost (so it seemed)
> Suspended by the blast that blew amain,
> Shouldering the naked crag.

The boys skated:—

> All shod with steel,
> We hissed along the polished ice in games
> Confederate, imitative of the chase
> And woodland pleasures,—the resounding horn,
> The pack loud chiming, and the hunted hare.

They played:—

From week to week, from month to month, we lived
A round of tumult. Duly were our games
Prolonged in summer till the daylight failed.

They boated:—

When summer came,
Our pastime was, on bright half-holidays,
To sweep along the plain of Windermere
With rival oars . . .

Miss Mason: Do we read that young Wordsworth had any experiences on horseback?

Miss Laurio: Yes, he did, when he and his schoolmates came back from their holidays with money in their pockets, and hired horses. Off they went, "proud to curb, and eager to spur on, the galloping steed"; and then he tells of their home-coming:—

Through the walls we flew
And down the valley, and, a circuit made
In wantonness of heart, through rough and smooth
We scampered homewards.

Miss Mason: Applause for Miss Laurio! That was quite complete. Although we cannot go back to those days of the late eighteenth century, and in some respects we would probably not wish to, it sounds like Wordsworth had a quite enviable childhood, at least in the sphere of *Dynamic Relations*. If some prophet had been able to look ahead and pick him out to his teachers or parents as one who would become famous for poems about clouds and daffodils, might that have changed the opportunities he was given, to one extreme or another?

Miss Bruce: I suppose that would depend on how they felt about clouds and daffodils.

[laughter]

Miss Bruce: No, what I mean is…if they did not care for that idea, they might have pushed him harder to do even more "manly" things, or put him in a military academy or some such. But if they did realize that his gift of writing was going to be very important, they might not have let him take as many chances as he did, hanging above ravens' nests and so on. Perhaps it's better that we don't know too early on what a child's particular strengths are going to be, or we might push them to specialize in one thing, or even push them out of an opportunity if it went against our plans for them.

Part Two

Miss Mason: Well, let us see if the same comparisons hold true as we examine *Affinity for Material*, the joy of handling natural materials and of making things from them. Miss Capehart, what were you able to find out about this?

Miss Capehart: Wordsworth says little about this, but Ruskin has more, probably because he had a stronger interest in art and design. Ruskin's "feelers" in this direction began with "two boxes of well-cut wooden bricks."

> I was afterwards (he says) gifted with a two-arched bridge, admirable in fittings of voussoir and keystone, and adjustment of the level courses of masonry with bevelled edges, into which they dovetailed in the style of Waterloo Bridge.

I had to look that up because I didn't know what voussoirs are. Do any of you know? No? They are the special blocks used to build arches, and keystones and springers are particular sorts of voussoirs.

Miss Mason: It appears that we all need to increase our affinity for building-bricks.

Miss Capehart: Anyway…

> Well-made centrings, and a course of inlaid steps down to the water, made this model largely, as accurately, instructive: and I was never weary of building, *un*-building–(it was too strong to be thrown down, but had always to be *taken* down) –and re-building it.

His friend and assistant William Gershom Collingwood later wrote that, while Ruskin liked to garden and wrote about botany, "yet in his practical gardening [he] was quite the landscapist. He liked making paths and contriving pretty nooks, building steps and bridges, laying out beds, woodcutting and so forth; but I never remember him potting and grafting and layering and budding; and as to the rarity of any plants in his garden, I believe he took far more pleasure in the wood-anemone—*Silvia*, he called it—than in anything buyable from the nurseryman's catalogue."

But if Ruskin had not, as a child, a wide acquaintance with the flowers of the field, he made up, perhaps, by the enormous attention he gave to such as came in his way; and, just as his bricks and his bridge gave him his initiation in the principles of architecture, so, perhaps, his early flower studies resulted in his power of seeing and expressing detail. He says of flowers, "My whole time passed in staring at them or into them…" This seems to have paid off, as later in life he was able to write these words to his art students:

> Suppose you have to paint the Narcissus of the Alps... First, you must outline its six petals, its central cup, and its bulbed stalk, accurately, in the position you desire. Then you must paint the cup of the yellow which is its yellow, and the stalk of the green which is its green, and the white petals of creamy white, not milky white. Lastly, you must modify these colours so as to make the cup look hollow and the petals bent; but, whatever shade you add must never destroy the impression, which is the first a child would receive from the flower, of its being a yellow, white and green thing, with scarcely

any shade in it.

Miss Mason: Miss White, you have also been studying Ruskin: have you anything to add about his early relations with nature?

Miss White: Yes, actually, he was quite interested in the study of minerals, beginning with river pebbles, and then as he explored around Matlock in Derbyshire, where his family stayed at a hotel. He wrote,

> In the glittering white broken spar, speckled with galena, by which the walks of the hotel garden were made bright, and in the slopes of the pretty village, and in many a happy walk along its cliffs, I pursued my mineralogical studies on fluor, calcite, and the ores of lead, and with indescribable rapture when I was allowed to go into a cave. My father and mother showed far more kindness than I knew, in yielding to my subterranean passion; for my mother could not bear dirty places, and my father had a nervous feeling that the ladders would break, or the roof fall, before we got out again. They went with me, nevertheless, wherever I wanted to go...

Later we find him going up Snowdon, "of which ascent I remember, as the most exciting event, the finding for the first time in my life a real 'mineral' for myself, a piece of copper pyrites!" This resulted in Ruskin's lifelong fascination with minerals, to which we owe *The Ethics of the Dust.*

Miss Mason: It may not be necessary to say much yet about Wordsworth's relations with nature, as this is so obvious from his poetry, and we will be discussing it in the next class. But was anyone able to discover if that affinity was discovered early on?

Miss Breckenridge: Wordsworth appears to have waited for his intimacy with wild-flowers until he could say of his sister Dorothy, "She gave me eyes, she gave me ears." Birds, as we have seen, he knew through that wicked joy of birds-nesting; but he also remembered that adventure on horseback to Furness Abbey, and the impression that a wren's singing made upon him there. But he himself seems to warn us about trying to pick out specific early influences too closely, or at least to say "this time was exactly where I got that idea," whether we are talking about our own memories, or trying to interest our children in some aspect of nature, or art, or history. Who hasn't taken children to a historic place, or to some great event, and seen them ignore whatever interested the adults, and notice only some obscure or even embarrassing point, such as whatever the monkeys were doing? But their later memories of that event may become part of a larger group of impressions that are just as important—do you see what I mean? So it's really not up to us as teachers to try to "class the cabinet / Of their sensations."

Miss Mason: And, as much the same could be said about *Education by Books*, that will be the topic of our next session.

Poetic Interlude #2

At the Sea-Side

by Robert Louis Stevenson

When I was down beside the sea
A wooden spade they gave to me
To dig the sandy shore.
My holes were empty like a cup.
In every hole the sea came up
Till it could come no more.

Personal Talk and Books

by William Wordsworth

Wings have we, and as far as we can go
We may find pleasure: wilderness and wood,
Blank ocean and mere sky, support that mood
Which with the lofty sanctifies the low:
Dreams, books, are each a world; and books, we know,
Are a substantial world, both pure and good:
Round these, with tendrils strong as flesh and blood,
Our pastime and our happiness will grow.
There find I personal themes, a plenteous store,
Matter wherein right voluble am I,
To which I listen with a ready ear.
Two shall be named, pre-eminently dear:—
The gentle Lady married to the Moor,
And heavenly Una with her milk-white Lamb.

Study 14: Insatiate Delight in Books

Prologue

Miss Mason: The idea that vivifies teaching in the Parents' Union is that "Education is the Science of Relations." But what do we mean by that?

We believe that children come into the world with a natural "appetency" for, and affinity with, all the material of knowledge; with interest in the heroic past and in the age of myths; a desire to know about everything that moves and lives, about strange places and strange peoples; a wish to handle material and to make; and a desire to run and ride and row and do whatever the law of gravitation permits.

Therefore we do not believe it is lawful for us, in the early days of a child's life, to select certain subjects for his education to the exclusion of others; to say he shall not learn Latin, for example, or shall not learn Science; but we endeavour that he shall have relations of pleasure and intimacy established with as many as possible of the interests proper to him; not learning a slight or incomplete smattering about this or that subject, but plunging into vital knowledge, with a great field before him which in all his life he will not be able to explore. In this conception we get that "touch of emotion" which vivifies knowledge, for it is probable that we *feel* only as we are brought into our proper vital relations.

A corollary of the principle that "education is the science of relations" is that no education seems to be worth the name which has not made children at home in the world of books, and so *related* them, mind to mind, with thinkers who have dealt with knowledge. We reject epitomes, compilations, and their like, and put into children's hands books which, long or short, are *living*. Thus it becomes a large part of the teacher's work to help children to deal with their books; so that the oral lesson and lecture are but small matters in education, and are used chiefly to summarize or to expand or illustrate.

Too much faith is commonly placed in oral lessons and lectures; "to be poured into like a bucket," as says Carlyle, "is not exhilarating to any soul"; neither is it exhilarating to have every difficulty explained to weariness, or to have the explanation teased out of one by questions. "I will not be put to the *question*. Don't you consider, sir, that these are not the manners of a gentleman? I will not be baited with *what* and *why*; what is this? what is that? why is a cow's tail long? why is a fox's tail bushy?" said Dr Johnson. This is what children think, though they say nothing. Oral lessons have their occasional use, and when they are fitly given it is the children who ask the questions. Perhaps it is not wholesome or quite honest for a teacher to pose as a source of all knowledge and to give "lovely" lessons. Such lessons are titillating for the moment, but they give children the minimum of mental labour, and the result is much the same as that left on older persons by the reading of a magazine *[Study 25]*.

Part One: Books

We find, on the other hand, that in working through a considerable book, which may take two or three years to master, the interest of boys and girls is well sustained to the end; they develop an intelligent curiosity as to causes and consequences, and are in fact educating themselves. We are told how Ruskin grew up upon Scott's *Waverley* novels, on Pope's Homer's *Iliad*, many of Shakespeare's plays, and much else that is delightful; but he does not give us an instance of the sort of thing we are looking for–the sudden keen, insatiate delight in a book which means kinship–until he is introduced to the poems and plays of Lord Byron. His first acquaintance with Byron he puts "about the beginning of the teen period":—

> ... by the end of this year 1834, I knew my Byron pretty well all through... So far as I could understand it, I rejoiced in all the sarcasm of *Don Juan*. But my firm decision, as soon as I got well into the later cantos of it, that Byron was to be my master in verse, as [much as William] Turner in colour, was made of course in that gosling (or say cygnet) epoch of existence, without consciousness of the deeper instincts that prompted it: only two things I consciously recognized, that his truth of observation was the most exact, and his chosen expression the most concentrated, that I had yet found in literature. . .But the thing wholly new and precious to me in Byron was his measured and living *truth*—measured, as compared with Homer; and living, as compared with everybody else . . . He taught me the meaning of Chillon and of Meillerie, and bade me seek first in Venice—the ruined homes of Foscari and Falieri Byron told me of, and reanimated for me, the real people whose feet had worn the marble I trod on.

There are several points there from which we might take suggestions. One is that we may not always realize ourselves how much weight, or how much meaning, lies behind an artist or writer for whom we feel an affinity; nor how much potential that relationship may have to change our own lives, or that of others. At the beginning, we may know only, like Ruskin, that we appreciate something specific about their style; or we may recognize, again like Ruskin to Lord Byron, some flash of essential truth, that has not surfaced as much with others. I earlier used the word "kinship," and that is similar to "kindred spirit"—someone or something for which we feel an instant affinity, a recognition that we seem to be of the same tribe.

And, as things have a tendency to do, that original affinity may wrap its arms and legs around new information, or spark new ideas. In Ruskin's case, Byron's descriptions of France and Italy increased his zeal to travel, and that formed a very important part of his own life and work. But we do not view the works of Byron as a sort of textbook or travel guide to be studied and quizzed, nor do we require our students to analyze his poems for examples of his "measured and living truth."

Miss White, will you tell us now about Wordsworth's affinity for books?

Miss White: He mentions reading *Don Quixote*, and there are a few other books which he seems to remember fondly. But the longest passage about books is about *The Arabian Nights*, or an extract from it, which made Wordsworth and his friend want to read more, so they saved their money, planning to buy all the volumes.

Through several months,
In spite of all temptation, we preserved
Religiously that vow; but firmness failed,
Nor were we ever masters of our wish.

Though they did not manage to buy those particular books, when he went back home during the school holidays, he was happy at least to find other good books he had left there. He writes that sometimes he would spend hours outdoors reading: even though the fishing was very good, the lure of the books was stronger.

And then there is this ode to romantic literature—not as in love stories, but the literary genre of Romance, medieval tales of chivalry. Considering that Wordsworth became a poet of the Romantic era, it makes sense that these "legends penned by dim light of monkish lamps" caught his imagination.

A gracious spirit o'er this earth presides,
And o'er the heart of man: invisibly
It comes, to works of unreproved delight,
And tendency benign, directing those
Who care not, know not, think not what they do.
The tales that charm away the wakeful night
In Araby romances; legends penned
For solace by dim light of monkish lamps;
Fictions, for ladies of their love, devised
By youthful squires; adventures endless, spun
By the dismantled warrior in old age,
Out of the bowels of those very schemes
In which his youth did first extravagate;
These spread like day, and something in the shape
Of these will live till man shall he no more.
Dumb yearnings, hidden appetites, are ours,
And they must have their food. Our childhood sits,
Our simple childhood, sits upon a throne
That hath more power than all the elements.

Miss Mason: Miss Breckenridge, will you continue?

Miss Breckenridge: I noticed this story of Wordsworth's first enthrallment by poetry:—

Twice five years
Or less I might have seen, when first my mind
With conscious pleasure opened to the charm
Of words in timeful order, found them sweet
For their own sakes, a passion and a power;
And phrases pleased me chosen for delight,
For pomp, or love. Oft, in the public roads
Yet unfrequented, while the morning light
Was yellowing the hill tops, I went abroad
With a dear friend, and for the better part
Of two delightful hours we strolled along
By the still borders of the misty lake,
Repeating favourite verses with one voice,
Or conning more, as happy as the birds
That round us chaunted.

Chosen for delight, for pomp, or for love: what a good way to describe a relationship with books!

Miss Mason: Thank you, Miss Breckenridge, well done. Now there is one "affinity" somewhat related to that of books, that we do not hear quite so much about, and that is what we call the *Historic Sense*, or what some would call the appreciation of the past. Now the awakening of the Historic Sense in Ruskin appears to be always–and here is a great lesson for us–connected with *places*; we may also note that historic interest and aesthetic delight are, for Ruskin, inseparable from each other. We have seen already how reading Byron served him in this way. Again, he tells us of the "three centres of my life's thought, Rouen, Geneva, and Pisa, which have been tutoresses of all I know and were mistresses of all I did from the first moments I entered their gates."

These came later, so are somewhat out of the scope of our discussion here; but he writes also about Abbeville, a place in France that he first visited in 1835, when he was about sixteen. Abbeville is the site of the Church of St. Wulfran, and over thirty years later Ruskin was still fascinated by what he called the "luscious richness" of its late Gothic style, especially when he compared it to the severity of some of the English church architecture. Because he *was* Ruskin, and liked to do the same thing in different ways, he wrote about Abbeville and the church; and painted it; and then displayed the painting along with some others while giving a lecture entitled "The Flamboyant Architecture of the Valley of the Somme," in 1869. He writes that Abbeville

> ...was entrance for me into immediately healthy labour and joy. . . .My most intense happinesses have of course been among mountains. But for cheerful, unalloyed, unwearying pleasure, the getting sight of Abbeville on a fine summer afternoon, jumping out in the courtyard of the Hotel de l'Europe and rushing down the street to see St. Wulfran again before the sun was off the towers, are things to cherish the past for—to the end.

"To the end"—what a beautiful summation of a lifelong affinity for a place!

However, it is true that our best educational seed may fall on a somewhat stony patch of ground in an otherwise fertile field. To be precise, I am speaking of a certain disconnection from the enjoyment of actual history, for both Ruskin and Wordsworth. Miss Capehart, what have you noticed about this?

Miss Capehart: Ruskin seemed to lack a real sense of living touch with the past, except as such touch was given by the newly discovered history of a place he happened to be in, as is shown in his first impressions of Rome:—

> We of course drove about the town, and saw the Forum, Coliseum, and so on. I had no distinct idea what the Forum was or ever had been, or how the three pillars, or the seven, were connected with it, or the Arch of Severus. . . What the Forum or Capitol had been, I did not in the least care; the pillars of the Forum I saw were on a small scale, and their capitals rudely carved, and the houses above them nothing like so interesting as the side of any close in the 'auld toun' of Edinburgh.

I suppose that may be somewhat of a relief to those of us whose students reading Plutarch cannot remember the difference between Timoleon and Themistocles, or where Macedonia was.

Miss Mason: Miss Laurio, will you continue with this topic, from your reading of Wordsworth?

Miss Laurio: Wordsworth, too, stood aloof from history. He was aware of

> Old, unhappy, far-off things
>
> And battles long ago;

but the past of nations did not enthrall him; even the throes of the French Revolution, to judge by what he tells us in the *Prelude*, hardly shook him to his foundation, though he took a walking tour on the Continent at the moment when, as he himself says—

> As if awaked from sleep, the nations hailed
>
> Their great expectancy.

But for him—

I looked upon these things
As from a distance; heard and saw and felt,
Was touched, but with no intimate concern...

So I guess we cannot all be historians, just as we are not all going to be scientists or linguists; but still it seems a bit sad that a deeper interest in human history was never quite awakened for either Wordsworth or Ruskin.

Miss Mason: Is it apparent that they were any more interested in their other school studies? Miss Glass?

Miss Glass: Ruskin gives us rather dry details of his experiences in Euclid, the Latin grammar, and the like, but neither boy appears to have been "stung with the rapture of a sudden thought" in the course of his lessons, unless Hawkshead Grammar School can take the credit for these lines:—

Many are the joys
Of youth, but oh! what happiness to live
When every hour brings palpable access
Of knowledge, when all knowledge is delight,
And sorrow is not there.

But the praise of the unfolding of the seasons follows, and I am afraid it is the lore *they* brought with them that Wordsworth had in his mind's eye, and not his school lessons.

Part Two: Other Relationships

Miss Mason: What about the human relationships we may build during our school days—the sense of *comradeship*? Indeed, this is something that is much touted by educators, including those who give prizes and scholarships. For example, one requirement of the Rhodes Scholarship it that the applicant must have "fellowship," or "instincts to lead and take an interest in his schoolmates." It is well that a talent for comradeship should be brought before us in this prominent way, as something truly vital: we do need to form close connections with others. But here is the rock upon which Ruskin's education split, as he was sadly aware; he never knew the joys of comradeship. Having spoken of "peace, obedience, faith; these three for chief good; next to these the habit of fixed attention with both eyes and mind," as the main blessings of his childhood, he goes on to enumerate "the equally dominant calamities":

> First, that I had nothing to love. My parents were–in a sort–visible powers of nature to me, no more loved than the sun and the moon: only I should have been annoyed and puzzled if either of them had

> gone out; (how much, now, when both are darkened!)—still less did I love God; not that I had any quarrel with Him, or fear of Him; but simply found what people told me was His service, disagreeable; and what people told me was His book, not entertaining. I had no companions to quarrel with neither; nobody to assist, and nobody to thank. Not a servant was ever allowed to do anything for me, but what it was their duty to do; and why should I have been grateful to the cook for cooking, or the gardener for gardening? . . . My present verdict, therefore, on the general tenor of my education at that time, must be, that it was at once too formal and too luxurious; leaving my character at the most important moment for its construction, cramped indeed, but not disciplined; and only by protection innocent, instead of by practice virtuous.

Cramped, but not disciplined; innocent by protection, but not virtuous by practice? Indeed, there is much of value to consider in those words; and we might find it equally valuable to turn them round, as a sort of child-raising motto: "Disciplined, but not cramped"; and "virtuous by practice, not only by protection."

Miss Bruce, can you describe the comradeship or other relationships in the life of Wordsworth?

Miss Bruce: Wordsworth, unlike Ruskin, lived the life of his school-fellows with entire *abandon*, and was rarely alone as a child. But besides that, he had a very strong sense from early on of who his "people" were. Sir Walter Scott claimed "intimacy with all ranks of my countrymen from the Scottish peer to the Scottish ploughman," and from that we get the *Waverley* novels. Wordsworth, on the other hand, felt kinship with the simple people of his "beloved Vale," and also with friends who shared his poetic interests, but he was not quite so curious about those beyond his own region or circle.

Miss Mason: Perhaps such limits contributed to the making of the poet of "Plain living and high thinking…" *[Wordsworth, "Written in London"]*. But such limitations may be hazardous; that is to say, we should not recommend that outlook for most children.

Miss Glass: I would like to say that it is difficult for some children to become the social creature that eases parents' and teachers' minds, and makes them think "oh, he'll be fine—look how he gets along with all his classmates." I recall as a child, going to the seaside with our relatives. I met another girl who was reading a book I liked, and we spent an enjoyable few minutes talking about our favourite scenes and so on; but my mother scolded me afterwards, and said my time should have been properly spent with my cousins, who, truth to tell, often led me into mischief. Should we push children into "comradeship" with those with whom they feel little affinity, or just the opposite, discourage them from friendships that we have not approved?

Miss Mason: As we have said before about the problems of arbitrary and legitimate authority: there is often a great need for fine discrimination in these matters. One child may certainly need to be pushed a little in the matter of developing friendships, because we know that such relationships are vital, that is, *vital* in the life-giving sense; and certainly we want our children to develop habits that make them able to be good friends, such as cheerfulness, loyalty, generosity, and so on. But as we also know that "children are born persons," we must also give respect to their individual temperaments, and allow them as much choice as possible in the matter of friendships.

We will end for now, but there will be one more talk about Wordsworth and Ruskin, and their example of the relationships and affinities that may be built up gradually, or discovered suddenly.

Study 15: In Which the Student Teachers Converse About Little Prigs, and Books, and Things

Miss Capehart: Did you know that in Shakespeare's time the word "prig" meant a "tinker" or "petty thief?": It wasn't until the next century that it started to mean…priggish. Like the little girl in the group who has to be the best-behaved, and she makes sure everyone knows it.

Miss Breckenridge: But there's a way of being priggish over one's education as well. I had this cousin named Eustace…horrible boy.

Miss Bruce: A model child who makes everyone else uncomfortable with his superiority.

Miss White: Or a wide-mouthed frog.

Miss Bruce: Say that again?

Miss White: There was this wide-mouthed frog, and she had babies, but she didn't know what to feed them.

Miss Bruce: But frogs don't feed their babies. This person needs more nature walks.

Miss White: Suspend your belief for a minute. So she went to the cow, and she said (stretching her mouth wide and speaking loudly), "Mrs. Cow, what do you feed your babies?" The cow said, "I feed my babies milk." The frog said (stretching her mouth wide and speaking loudly), "Oh, that's nice." And she went on to the horse. She said (stretching her mouth wide and speaking loudly), "Mrs. Horse, what do you feed your babies?" The horse said, "I feed them hay." The frog said (stretching her mouth wide and speaking loudly), "Oh, that's nice." Finally she came to a very big snake. She said (stretching her mouth wide and speaking loudly), "Mrs. Snake, what do you feed your babies?" The snake said, "I feed them wide-mouthed frogs." The frog said (pursing up her mouth and whispering), "Oh—that's nice."

[laughter]

Miss Laurio: Well, I've known a few wide-mouthed frogs. Dear Miss Glass, you are awfully quiet with your nose in that book—do you have something you wish to share with the class?

Miss Glass: It's something in *The Prelude*. Wordsworth was pretty satisfied with his free-roaming childhood, and he says here that he can't resist adding a few comments and thanking the powers that be that he was "reared / Safe from an evil which these days have laid / Upon the children of the land, a pest / That might have dried me up, body and soul." He talks about his mother, because he thinks that she did things the right way, that she:

> Was not puffed up by false unnatural hopes,
> Nor selfish with unnecessary cares,
> Nor with impatience from the season asked
> More than its timely produce; rather loved
> The hours for what they are, than from regard
> Glanced on their promises in restless pride.

Miss Breckenridge: Loving the hours for what they are: I like that.

Miss Glass: So then there's this on his view of the modern child, and I think this is a bit like your wide-mouthed frog:

> Full early trained to worship seemliness,
> This model of a child is never known
> To mix in quarrels; that were far beneath
> Its dignity; with gifts he bubbles o'er
> As generous as a fountain; selfishness
> May not come near him, nor the little throng
> Of flitting pleasures tempt him from his path...

Miss Laurio: Sounds like a regular modern major general.

Miss Glass: And a little further on:

> Yet innocent himself withal, though shrewd,
> And can read lectures upon innocence;

A miracle of scientific lore,
Ships he can guide across the pathless sea,
And tell you all their cunning; he can read
The inside of the earth, and spell the stars;
He knows the policies of foreign lands;
Can string you names of districts, cities, towns,
The whole world over, tight as beads of dew
Upon a gossamer thread; he sifts, he weighs;
All things are put to question; he must live
Knowing that he grows wiser every day
Or else not live at all, and seeing too
Each little drop of wisdom as it falls
Into the dimpling cistern of his heart:
For this unnatural growth the trainer blame,
Pity the tree.

Miss Bruce: Indeed.

Miss Glass: Oh, and here's the curriculum for the Wordsworth Primary School.

Meanwhile old grandame earth is grieved to find
The playthings, which her love designed for him,
Unthought of: in their woodland beds the flowers
Weep, and the river sides are all forlorn.
Oh! give us once again the wishing cap
Of Fortunatus, and the invisible coat
Of Jack the Giant-killer, Robin Hood,
And Sabra in the forest with St. George!
The child, whose love is here, at least, doth reap
One precious gain, that he forgets himself.

[bell ringing]

Miss White: Time to go for Swedish Drill with Miss Duran.

[much bustling and putting on of shawls]

Miss Glass: Wait, what? Oh my, girls, I just discovered something important here. Don't go…All right, fine, I'll read it on the way.

Tamed to their bidding; they who have the skill
To manage books, and things, and make them act
On infant minds as surely as the sun
Deals with a flower; the keepers of our time,
The guides and wardens of our faculties,

Miss Capehart: Oh, not the faculties again. Look, there goes a hawk.

Miss Glass: But did you notice? "Books, and things."

Sages who in their prescience would control
All accidents, and to the very road
Which they have fashioned would confine us down,
Like engines; when will their presumption learn,
That in the unreasoning progress of the world
A wiser spirit is at work for us,
A better eye than theirs, most prodigal
Of blessings, and most studious of our good,
Even in what seem our most unfruitful hours?

Miss White: Swedish Drill is not exactly my most fruitful hour.

Miss Capehart: Well, wiser spirits have decided.

Miss Glass:

A race of real children; not too wise,
Too learned, or too good; / but wanton, fresh,
And bandied up and down by love and hate;
Not unresentful where self-justified;
Fierce, moody, patient, venturous, modest, shy;
Mad at their sports like withered leaves in winds;
Though doing wrong and suffering, and full oft
Bending beneath our life's mysterious weight
Of pain, and doubt, and fear, yet yielding not
In happiness to the happiest upon earth.
Simplicity in habit, truth in speech,
Be these the daily strengtheners of their minds;
May books and Nature be their early joy!

> And knowledge, rightly honoured with that name —
>
> Knowledge not purchased by the loss of power!

Miss Laurio: Simplicity in habit, truth in speech.

Miss Breckenridge: And power over oneself. Yes, we get it.

Miss Bruce: And Miss Mason obviously did too.

Study 16: Vocation

The student teachers return to the lecture room for a final talk drawn from the writings of Wordsworth and Ruskin.

Part One

Miss Mason: We might trace the consummation of various other affinities in our two illustrious subjects, but time fails; I can only indicate the joy of pursuing the acquaintanceship, followed by the endless occupation for mind and heart, in that high intimacy which we call the *Vocation* of each of these men of genius. By *Vocation* we mean not only occupation, but calling; not just our daily work, but our life's work. What is it that inspires the discovery of our own piece of work to do in the world?

As you students have given your all in the previous sessions, I will ask you this time only to listen and consider carefully. We will begin with Ruskin.

Ruskin's family, if this has not already been made clear, was of the newly emerging "middle class"; they had money, and they also valued education. His father owned many books and collected watercolour paintings by British artists of the time. His mother would have preferred he go into the church, but his father didn't seem to mind what profession he followed, as long as it wasn't one of the "trades." When young John was ten years old, his father sent him a letter which included these words:

> You are blessed with a fine Capacity & even Genius & you owe it as a Duty to the author of your Being & the giver of your Talents to cultivate your powers & to use them in his Service & for the benefit of your fellow Creatures. You may be doomed to enlighten a People by your Wisdom & to adorn an age by your learning.

Ruskin's "career" began when, on his thirteenth birthday (or thereabouts), his father's business partner, Mr. Henry Telford, gave him a copy of Rogers' *Italy*, of which he says "I took [the Turner vignettes] for my only masters, and set myself to imitate them as far as I possibly could by fine pen shading. . ."

For those of us of a later period, Ruskin's brief description of his birthday gift may not make much of an impression. If you will forgive a brief veering off from our subject, we should begin with the poet, Samuel Rogers, who lived from 1763 to 1855. Rogers was a celebrated poet and social celebrity in his day, a friend and colleague of the Romantic poets. Well, in 1814, Rogers was touring Europe, keeping a diary of everything he saw; and the biggest event was that, just as he reached Naples, the news of Napoleon's escape from Elba forced him to return to England. A few years later, he published a book-length poem based on his trip, called *Italy*. But the poem was not an immediate success, so Rogers enlarged and revised it; and then he had the inspiration to add illustrations. He commissioned watercolours from three artists, one of whom was J.M.W. Turner, and these were added as steel engravings to the 1830 edition of his book. This time it was a great success, and he was even invited to succeed Wordsworth as Poet Laureate.

So then to the pictures that so inspired Ruskin. Turner himself had visited Italy in 1819; but he combined his own memories of the "modern" country there with its ancient past, as he had seen it in art and monuments. He painted them as watercolours, but Rogers' readers had to be content for that time with the black and white versions that were scattered quite lavishly through the book. Studying these gave Ruskin, first of all, a wonderful start at that thing which many call a "career," but which we prefer to think of as his *vocation*; and, second, a lifelong appreciation for the work of Turner. He writes about his own purchase of Turner's watercolour "Harlech":

> Whatever germs of better things remained in me, were then all centred in this love of Turner. It was not a piece of painted paper, but a Welsh castle and village, and Snowdon in blue cloud, that I bought for my seventy pounds.

In your reading of *Praeterita*, you will no doubt have come across Ruskin's descriptions of his own attempts at drawing from nature, but time prevents us from going into them now, except for this very interesting paragraph:

> I took out my book and began to draw a little aspen tree, on the other side of the cart road, carefully. . . Languidly, but not idly, I began to draw it; and as I drew, the languor passed away, the beautiful lines insisted on being traced, without weariness. More and more beautiful they became as each rose out of the rest and took its place in the air. With wonder increasing every instant, I saw that they composed themselves by finer laws than any known of men. At last the tree was there, and everything that I had thought before about trees nowhere. . . "He hath made everything beautiful in His time" became for me thenceforward the interpretation of the bond between the human mind and all visible things.

"Everything that I had thought before about trees [was] nowhere." Ruskin *knew* those trees, knew them in an entirely new way, through his drawing of them. The relationship had been established forever.

Part Two

Miss Mason: We have seen in Ruskin and Wordsworth the strenuous attention–the condition of receptiveness–which made each of them a producer after his kind; and whosoever will play the game, whether it be cricket or portrait painting, must learn the rules with all diligence and get skill by his labour. It is true, as Macbeth says, "the labour we delight in physics pain," but it is also true that we cannot catch hold of any one of the affinities that are in waiting for us without strenuous effort and without reverence. A London bird-lover, one would say, has chosen for himself an easy joy; but no: your true bird-lover is out of doors by four in the morning to assist at the *levée* of the birds; nay, is he not in Hyde Park by 2:30 a.m. to see—the kingfisher, no less! He lies in wait in secret places to watch the goings on of the feathered peoples, travels far afield to make a new acquaintance in the bird-world; in fact, gives to the study of birds attention, labour, love, and reverence. He gets joy in return, so is perhaps little conscious of effort; but the effort is made all the same.

How shall we venture to trace the growth of that austere, most gracious and enthralling intimacy with Nature which was to Wordsworth the master-light of all his seeing? He unfolds to us—

> The simple ways in which my childhood walked;
> Those chiefly that first led me to the love
> Of rivers, woods, and fields. The passion yet
> Was in its birth, sustained as might befall
> By nourishment that came unsought.

We cannot trace every step of the growth of this ethereal passion, but only take a phase of it here and there. The boy and some of his schoolfellows were boating on Windermere in the late evening:—

> —and the sky,
> Never before so beautiful, sank down
> Into my heart, and held me like a dream!
> Thus were my sympathies enlarged, and thus
> Daily the common range of visible things
> Grew dear to me: already I began
> To love the sun; a boy, I loved the sun,
> Not as I since have loved him, as a pledge
> And surety of our earthly life, a light
> Which we behold and feel we are alive;
> Not for his bounty to so many worlds—
> But for this cause, that I had seen him lay

His beauty on the morning hills, had seen

The western mountain touch his setting orb.

"Thus were my sympathies enlarged." "Thus daily the common range of visible things grew dear to me." And why does Wordsworth say, particularly, that he loved the sun? Because he had *seen* "him lay / His beauty on the morning hills."

We are steadfast to the affinities we take hold of, till death do us part, or longer. Because, as we must always remember:

Everyone: Education is the Science of Relations.

Part Three

Miss Mason: We may take one more look at this marvellous boy, who, become a man, held that *every* child, as he, is born a poet. Wordsworth speaks here of being in his seventeenth year. As this passage is a bit longer, I will pass the book around, and we will take turns reading. Miss Laurio, will you begin here?

Miss Laurio:

Thus while the days flew by, and years passed on,

From nature and her overflowing soul

I had received so much, that all my thoughts

Were steeped in feeling;

Miss Glass:

I was only then

Contented, when with bliss ineffable

I felt the sentiment of Being spread

O'er all that moves and all that seemeth still;

O'er all that, lost beyond the reach of thought

And human knowledge, to the human eye

Invisible, yet liveth to the heart;

Miss Capehart:

O'er all that leaps and runs, and shouts and sings,

Or beats the gladsome air; o'er all that glides

Beneath the wave, yea, in the wave itself,

And mighty depth of waters.

Miss Mason: Miss Bruce, will you continue from this place I have marked?

Miss Bruce:

...if I should fail, with grateful voice
To speak of you, Ye Mountains and Ye Lakes,
And sounding Cataracts! Ye Mists and Winds
That dwell among the hills where I was born.
If, in my youth, I have been pure in heart,
If, mingling with the world, I am content
With my own modest pleasures, and have liv'd,
With God and Nature communing, remov'd
From little enmities and low desires,
The gift is yours;

Miss White:

if in these times of fear,
This melancholy waste of hopes o'erthrown,
If, 'mid indifference and apathy
And wicked exultation, when good men,
On every side fall off we know not how,
To selfishness, disguis'd in gentle names
Of peace, and quiet, and domestic love,
Yet mingled, not unwillingly, with sneers
On visionary minds;

Miss Breckenridge:

if in this time
Of dereliction and dismay, I yet
Despair not of our nature; but retain
A more than Roman confidence, a faith
That fails not, in all sorrow my support,
The blessing of my life, the gift is yours...

Miss Mason:

> Ye mountains! thine, O Nature! Thou hast fed
> My lofty speculations; and in thee,
> For this uneasy heart of ours I find
> A never-failing principle of joy,
> And purest passion.

I cannot stop here to gather any more of the instruction and edification contained in those two great educational books. It is enough for now if they have shown us in what manner children attach themselves to their proper affinities, given opportunity and liberty. Our part is to drop occasion freely in the way, whether in school or at home.

Part Four

Miss Mason: Neither *The Prelude* nor *Praeterita* lends itself to the study of the highest Relationship, the profoundest Intimacy, which awaits the soul of man; so we must go elsewhere for examples of this. Think of those people you have known who have seemed to most deeply desire an intimate relationship with God. Have you read of Brother Lawrence, a lay Brother among the barefooted Carmelites, whose story is told in *The Practice of the Presence of God?*

His biographer writes this:

> The first time I saw Brother Lawrence was upon the 3rd of August, 1666. He told me that God had done him a singular favour in his conversion at the age of eighteen. That in the winter, seeing a tree stripped of its leaves, and considering that within a little time the leaves would be renewed, and after that the flower and fruit appear, he received a high view of the Providence and Power of God, which has never since been effaced from his soul.
>
> That this view had perfectly set him loose from the world, and kindled in him such a love for God, that he could not tell whether it had increased in about forty years that he had lived since.
>
> That he had been footman to M. Fieubert, the treasurer, and that he was a great awkward fellow who broke everything.
>
> That he had desired to be received into a monastery, thinking he would there be made to smart for his awkwardness and the faults he should commit, and so he should sacrifice to God his life, with its pleasures: but that God had disappointed him, he having met with nothing but satisfaction in that state...

Now you may have read those famous lines about Brother Lawrence that tell about his praying among the pots and pans, which some have misinterpreted to mean that God does not expect busy people to take actual time on their knees. But listen to these words, that I believe better demonstrate his great sense of intimacy and joy in the divine Relationship.

> That with him the set times of prayer were not different from other times; that he retired to pray according to the directions of his Superior, but that he did not want such retirement, nor ask for it, because his greatest business did not divert him from God...
>
> That the greatest pains or pleasures of this world were not to be compared with what he had experienced of both kinds in a spiritual state; so that he was careful for nothing and feared nothing, desiring but one only thing of God, viz., that he might not offend Him...
>
> When outward business diverted him a little from the thought of God, a fresh remembrance coming from God invested his soul, and so inflamed and transported him that it was difficult for him to contain himself, that he was more united to God in his outward employments than when he left them for devotion in retirement.

Thank you for your attention, and I wish you all success in your educational endeavours. The gift is yours.

Notes for a New Era

Where did you come from?

If you were writing your own autobiography, in verse or prose, what evidence would you include of your "early affinities?" Were they given to you purposely (such as music lessons), or did they happen accidentally?

Other Biographies

Miss Mason chose to study Wordsworth and Ruskin, partly because they were able to describe their own stories in a literary style, but also because neither of them described their childhoods as "perfect." Choose an (auto)biography of someone that is of interest to you, and search out (as the students did) how your subject did or did not experience early opportunities to connect with nature, with books, with other people, and so on; and, if possible, how that affected him or her later on. Were there certain events that sparked an interest—in the case of a musician, for example, the gift of an instrument? Or a teacher who encouraged those affinities? Was there some object that they cherished as a representation of those early awakenings?

Three Instruments

> Parents and teachers should know how to make sensible use of a child's **circumstances** (*atmosphere*) to forward his sound education; should train him in the *discipline* of the **habits** of the good life; and should *nourish his life* with **ideas**, the food upon which personality waxes strong. These three we believe to be the *only* instruments of which we may make lawful use in the upbringing of children; and any short cut we take by trading on their sensibilities, emotions, desires, or passions, will bring us and our children to grief.

These instruments represent external factors (like the outer parts of a cell), and are therefore accessible and legitimate to us; the internal factors are the ones with which we must not meddle. The "curriculum" or "syllabus" application of this will be examined more deeply in the sections to come. But in the meantime, we have covered the first twelve principles of education (see the Appendices)! And it is *because* we believe that children are born persons, and that the principles of authority and obedience are natural and necessary, that we turn to atmosphere, discipline and living ideas as both the limits and the possibilities of education.

Here is something to consider (a look ahead): is there one or the other of these three instruments that you find easy and natural to work with; or one that pushes you in uncomfortable directions? Later in the book, Miss Mason points out that different cultures and eras may draw on one of the three, and neglect the others. What problems might occur if the instruments got out of balance?

The "Slow" Movement

Miss Mason recommended a "steady unruffled course of work" as sufficient to offset a lack of extracurricular activities and classes, and suggested that such a lifestyle might even be the preferred one for the building of various affinities. Do you agree?

Leaping and Riding

> All children should have relations with earth and water, should run and leap, ride and swim, should establish the relation of maker to material in as many kinds as may be...

If you are teaching or caring for children—or other people—which of the relations listed do they have the fullest opportunity to develop? Which ones are there, but to a lesser extent? Which ones not at all? Is there anything you can do to remedy that?

Wordsworth's Mother

> Was not puffed up by false unnatural hopes,
> Nor selfish with unnecessary cares,
> Nor with impatience from the season asked
> More than its timely produce; rather loved
> The hours for what they are, than from regard
> Glanced on their promises in restless pride.

As a teacher, caregiver, or in your own life, how are you "loving the hours for what they are?"

Part Four: Setting Their Feet (The Interviewer Returns)

We believe that the ignorance of children is illimitable, but that, on the other hand, their intelligence is hardly to be reckoned with by our slower wits. (*School Education*, p. 223)

Our concern is to give children such knowledge as shall open up for them as large a share as may be of the world they live in for their use and enjoyment. (*School Education*, p. 225)

The people are reasonably content with plain sense; they are better pleased with sound sense dressed with learning or ample experience. If to this is added wit and fancy, they repay all that with proper appreciation. And if the whole be inspired with a deep moral impulse, and breathe the breath of a noble heart, every one recognizes that too... If a lecture is but interesting in the delivery, and full of meat afterwards for a whole week's picking, it sits in judgment on another lecture, brilliant in delivery, but leaving no permanent impressions, no questions, no facts, no reasonings, for after-discussions. It does not take a community long to perceive that some lectures instruct them wearisomely, that some instruct and inspire, that some inspire but do not instruct, that some, like fire-works, are magnificent while going off and nothing afterwards, and others, like a pomological show, are fine in the exhibition, and very juicy and refreshing afterwards. (Henry Ward Beecher, *Eyes and Ears*)

Study 17: School-Books, or School Books?

Miss Hagan returns to Miss Mason's study, with the purpose of finding out more about the PNEU, particularly on the topic of school-books and how they "make for education."

Part One

Miss Hagan: What is the purpose of the Parents' Union?

Miss Mason: Our aim in education is to give children vital interests in as many directions as possible—to set their feet in a large room (Psalm 31:8)—because the crying evil of the day is, it seems to me, intellectual inanition. Inanition has two meanings: exhaustion caused by malnourishment, or a lack of mental vigour and spiritual enthusiasm. Children suffering from this have little or no healthy curiosity, power of attention, or of effort; what is worse, they lose spontaneity and initiative; they expect life to drop into them like drops into a rain-tub, without effort or intention on their part. If we, as educators, believe that a young person, of any walk of life, is in the world to lay hold of all he can of those possessions which endure; that full, happy living, expansion, expression, resourcefulness, power of initiative, serviceableness—in a word, *character*, for him, depends upon how far he apprehends the relationships proper to him and how many of them he seizes—if this is our contention, then we should be gravely uneasy when his education leaves him (or her) with prejudices rather than real concern for others; and caring for "events" (in the sporting sense) rather than having interests and pursuits.

Miss Hagan: Do you find that young people generally are lacking principles?

Miss Mason: You are expecting me to say yes to that, of course, perhaps because I am getting old and that is the sort of thing every old person says. And perhaps I should not argue with it entirely. But I believe that the best of our young people do have principles; they bring them away from their schools fully as much as from their homes. Our educational shortcomings seem to be *intellectual* rather than *moral.*

We have been made familiar with the phrase "educational unrest," and we all feel its fitness. Never were there more able and devoted teachers, whether as the heads or on the staffs of schools of all classes. Money, labour, and research are freely spent on education, theory is widely studied, and pains are taken to learn what is done elsewhere; yet there is something amiss beyond that "divine discontent" which leads to effort. We know that a change of front is necessary; and we are ready, provided that the change be something more than an experiment. Headmasters and mistresses are, I believe, amongst the persons most ready to fall in with a sound reform; but, because these are persons with wide experience and highly-trained intellects, they are unwilling to launch changes which have not a philosophic basis as well as a utilitarian end.

Miss Hagan: Should education not be adapted to the child-mind?

Miss Mason: There is no such thing. The fact is, we undervalue children. The notion that an infant is a huge "oyster," who by slow degrees, and more and more, develops into that splendid intellectual and moral being, a full-grown man or woman, has been impressed upon us so much of late years that we believe intellectual spoon-meat to be the only food for what we are pleased to call "little minds." It is nothing to us that William Morris read his first *Waverley* novel when he was four and had read the whole series by the time he was seven. Thomas Babington Macaulay seems to have begun life as a great reader. We know the delightful story of how, when Hannah More called on his parents, he, a little boy of four, came forward with pretty hospitality to say that if she "would be good enough to come in" he would bring her "a glass of old spirits." He explained afterwards that "Robinson Crusoe often had some."

Miss Hagan: That's very funny.

Miss Mason: I was just reading something else about Macaulay; oh yes, here it is.

> About this period his father took him on a visit to Lady Waldegrave at Strawberry Hill, and was much pleased to exhibit to his old friend the fair bright boy, dressed in a green coat with red collar and cuffs, a frill at the throat, and white trousers. After some time had been spent among the wonders of the Orford collection, of which he ever afterwards carried a catalogue in his head, a servant who was waiting upon the company in the great gallery spilt some hot coffee over his legs. The hostess was all kindness and compassion, and when, after a while, she asked how he was feeling, the little fellow looked up in her face and replied: "Thank you madam, the agony is abated." [Trevelyan's *Life and Letters of Lord Macaulay*]

In practical working we find this idea a great power; the teachers do not talk down to the children; they are careful not to explain every word that is used, or to ascertain if children understand every detail. Not what we have learned, but what we are waiting to know is the delectable part of knowledge. Nor should knowledge be "peptonized" or diluted, but offered to the children with some substance in it and some vitality. We find that children can cover a large and various field with delight and intelligence in the time that is usually wasted over "the three R's," object-lessons, and other much-diluted matter in which the teaching is more than the knowledge.

Miss Hagan: You speak of teaching that is more than knowledge; is there knowledge that is more than teaching?

Miss Mason: The distinction between *knowledge* and *information* is, I think, fundamental. Information is the record of facts, experiences, appearances, etc., whether in books or in the verbal memory of the individual. Knowledge, it seems to me, implies the result of the voluntary and delightful action of the mind upon the material presented to it. Great minds, a Darwin or a Plato, are able to deal at first hand with appearances or experiences; the ordinary mind gets a little of its knowledge by such direct dealing, but for the most part it is set in action by the vivifying knowledge of others, which is at the same time a stimulus and a point of departure. The *information* acquired in the course of education is only by chance, and here and there, of practical value. *Knowledge*, on the other hand–that is, the product of the vital action of the mind on the material presented to it–*is power*; as it implies an increase of intellectual aptitude in new directions, and an always new point of departure.

Perhaps the chief function of a teacher is to distinguish information from knowledge in the acquisitions of his pupils. Because knowledge *is* power, the child who has got knowledge will certainly *show* power in dealing with it. He will recast, condense, illustrate, or narrate with vividness and with freedom the arrangement of his words. The child who has got only information will write and speak in the stereotyped phrases of his text-book, or will mangle in his notes the words of his teacher.

Miss Hagan: Let me ask you, what subjects are most important for children to study?

Miss Mason: Perhaps the main part of a child's education should be concerned with the great human relationships. History, Literature, Art, Languages (ancient or modern), Travel—all of these are the record or expression of persons; so is Science, so far as it is the history of discoveries, the record of observations; that is, so far as it is to be got out of *Books*. Essentially, however, Science falls under the heading of *Education by Things*, and is too large a subject for us to deal with here.

Before all these ranks Religion, including our relations of worship, loyalty, love and service to God; and next in order, perhaps, the intimate interpersonal relations implied in such terms as Self-knowledge, Self-control *[Study 26]*.

Knowledge in all these various fields is due to children; for there seems reason to believe that the limit to human *intelligence* coincides with the limit to human *interests*; in fact, we may say that a normal person of poor and narrow intelligence is so because the interests proper to him have not been called into play. The curriculum which should give children their due therefore falls into some six or eight groups—Religion, Philosophy (of the sort that I just mentioned), History, Languages, Mathematics, Science, Art, Physical Exercises, and Manual Crafts.

Study 18: Choosing Books

Miss Mason: The great educational failure we have still to deal with is in the matter of *Books*. We know that *Books* store the knowledge and thought of the world; but the mass of knowledge, the multitude of books, overpower us, and we think we may select here and there, from this book and that, fragments and facts of knowledge, to be dealt out, whether in the little cram book or the oral lesson.

Miss Hagan: So…how do school-books make for education? And do we need to use a hyphen there? Is there a difference between school books and school-books?

Miss Mason: Sir Philip Magnus says, speaking of the schools of the future:—

> We shall no longer require children to learn by constant repetition, scraps of history, geography, and grammar, nor try to teach them fragments of so-called science...The main feature of the reading lesson will be to show the use books, how they may be consulted to ascertain what other people have said or done, and how they be read for the pleasure they afford. The storing of the memory with facts is no part of elementary school work...It is not enough that a child should learn how to write, he must know what to write. He must learn to describe clearly what he has heard or seen, to transfer to written language his sense-impressions, and to express concisely his own thoughts.

And of course we emphasize the *habit* of reading as a chief acquirement of school life. It is only those who have read who do read. But, all in all, Sir Philip does agree with much of our own thought.

Now, school-books, with a hyphen, might imply little "readers" and compendiums; books produced for use in schools, for which we have occasionally found use, because "all is fish that comes to our net"; but we have thrown many of those back in the water. But "school books," without a hyphen, might be any very good books from which children are expected to read and learn, in the classroom or out of it; or I suppose they might as equally be bad books. This book I will use as an example is a Swedish novel, from many years ago, so not a school book itself; but it contains a passage concerning the power of what we may assume are school-books, with a hyphen—but very good school-books.

Miss Hagan: *[scribbling] The Neighbours*, by Frederika Bremer. You said it's a novel?

Miss Mason: It may be somewhat autobiographical as well. Well, I cannot read you the whole incident now, but I will try to summarize. Our narrator recalls that, at the age of sixteen, she had trouble with one of her shoulders, and her parents sent her to a class of gymnastic exercise, in a room equipped with "ropes, ladders and poles," where she was given training in "the bending of the back" and "exercises of the arms and legs." There seems to have been quite a large group of girls taking part, and although the narrator says that she was a little shy at first, before the end of the second week she had become the leader of her class. She writes:

> At that time I was studying Greek history; their heroes and their heroic deeds filled my imagination even in the gymnastic school. I proposed to my band to assume masculine and antique names and, in this place, to answer to no other than such as Agamemnon,

> Epaminondas, etc. For myself I chose the name of Orestes, and called my best friend in the class, Pylades. There was a tall thin girl, with a Finlandish accent, whom I greatly disliked, chiefly on account of the disrespect for me and my ideas which she manifested without reserve;...from this arose fresh cause for quarrels.
>
> Although in love with the Greek history, I was no less taken with the Swedish. Charles XII. was my idol, and I often entertained my friends in my class with narration of his deeds till my own soul was on fire with the most glowing enthusiasm. Like a shower of cold water, Darius (the tall girl, whose name was Britsa) one day came into the midst of us, and opposed me with the assertion that the Czar Peter I. was a much greater man than Charles XII.

So the two girls argued over it, throwing facts of history in each other's faces, until finally our narrator challenged the girl she called Darius to a fight with fencing swords, to defend the honour of their heroes.

> Darius and I saluted each other proudly and distantly. I gave her the first choice of the swords. She took one and flourished it about quite dexterously, as if she had been accustomed to the use of it. I saw myself (in imagination) already stabbed to the heart...'Czar Peter *was* a great man,' cried Darius. 'Down with him! long life to Charles XII!' I cried, bursting into a furious rage. I placed myself in an attitude of defence. Darius did the same...Our swords clashed one against the other, and in the next moment I was disarmed and thrown on the ground. Darius stood over me and I believed my last hour had arrived. How astonished was I, however, when my enemy threw her sword away from her, took me by the hand and lifted me up, whilst she cheerfully cried: 'Well, now you have satisfaction; let us be good friends again; you are a brave little body!' At this moment a tremendous noise was heard at the door and in rushed the fencing master and three teachers. My senses now forsook me.

Miss Hagan: She fainted? And what happened after that?

Miss Mason: It took her several weeks in bed to recover, and she admits that the incident "cooled her violent temperament." But here is the question we need to ask: how did the girls get their enthusiasm? What was it, we wonder, in their school-books that they found so exciting? And we must assume that it was, indeed, their school-books, as the oral lesson for young children, and the lecture for older ones, had not been invented at that time. We certainly use books in our English schoolrooms today; but one does not hear of wild enthusiasm, ungovernable excitement, over the tabulated events of the history books, the tabulated facts of the science "primers" or "readers." Those Swedish girls must have used books of another sort; and it is to our interest to find out of what sort.

Miss Hagan: Is there a record of what books they used?

Miss Mason: No; for that, we must look for information to the girls themselves. We cannot summon them to give a direct answer, but if we can get at what they *were*, we shall be able to make a good guess at what should fire their souls.

Miss Hagan: And what was that?

Miss Mason: The story discloses no more than that they were *intelligent* girls, probably the children of intelligent parents. But that is enough for our purpose. The question rather resolves itself into—What manner of book will find its way with upheaving effect into the mind of an intelligent boy or girl? The question is not what the girl or boy *likes*, such as the twaddle of goody-goody story books, or the condiments of highly-spiced tales of adventure. We are all capable of *liking* mental food of a poor quality and a titillating nature; and possibly such food is good for us when our minds are in need of an elbow-chair; but our spiritual life is sustained on other stuff, whether we be children or adults. (By "spiritual" I mean that which is not corporeal; and which, for the sake of convenience, we call by various names—the life of thought, the life of feeling, the life of the soul.)

But it is curious how every inquiry, superficial as it may seem to begin with, leads us to fundamental principles. This simple-seeming question—what manner of school-books should our boys and girls use?—leads us straight to one of the two great principles of educational thought.

Miss Hagan: Which is…

Miss Mason: I will come back to that in a minute. We still need to answer the question, "what manner of school books?" The power of giving impulse and stirring emotion is another benefit of books, the *right* books; but that is just the question–which *are* the right books? Well, that is a point upon which I should not wish to play "Sir Oracle." The "hundred best books for the schoolroom" *may* be put down on a list, but not by me. I venture to propose one or two principles in the matter of school-books, and shall leave the far more difficult part, the application of those principles, to your readers.

And in the same way, I think we owe it to children to let them dig their knowledge, of whatever subject, for themselves out of the fit book; and there are two reasons for this. What a child *digs for* is his own possession; what is poured into his ear, like the idle song of a pleasant singer, floats out as lightly as it came in, and is rarely assimilated. Do you know that children's rhyme that goes,

> Said the first little chicken,
> With a strange little squirm,
> "I wish I could find
> A fat little worm."

Said the second little chicken,
With an odd little shrug,
"I wish I could find
A fat little bug."

Said the third little chicken,
With a sharp little squeal,
"I wish I could find
Some nice yellow meal..."

"Now see here," said the mother,
From the green garden patch,
"If you want any breakfast,
Just come here and SCRATCH!"

I do not mean to say that the lecture and the oral lesson are without their uses; but these uses are, to give impulse and to *order* knowledge; and not to convey knowledge, or to afford us that part of our education which comes of fit knowledge, fitly given.

I believe that spiritual life, using *spiritual* in the sense I have indicated, is sustained upon only one manner of diet–the diet of ideas–the living progeny of living minds. If ideas must reach us directly from the mind of the thinker, then it is chiefly by means of the books they have written that we get into touch with the best minds. Now, if we send to any publisher for his catalogue of school books–that is, school-books with a hyphen–we find that it is accepted as the nature of a school-book that it be drained dry of living thought. It may bear the name of a thinker, but often it is the abridgment of an abridgment, and all that is left for the unhappy scholar is the dry bones of his subject, denuded of soft flesh and living colour, of the stir of life and power of moving. Nothing is left but what Oliver Wendell Holmes calls the "mere brute fact."

It cannot be too often said that information is not education, and instruction is not education [*Study 24*]. You may answer an examination question about the position of the Seychelles and the Comoro Islands without having been anywise nourished by the fact of these island groups existing in such and such latitudes and longitudes; but if you follow Frank T. Bullen and his whaling adventures in *The Cruise of the Cachalot*, the names excite that little mental stir which indicates the reception of real knowledge. Here, perhaps you could read some of it aloud.

Miss Hagan:

> We did not court danger by hugging too closely any of the ugly reefs and banks that abound in this notably difficult strait, but gave them all a respectfully wide berth. It was a feature of our navigation that, unless we had occasion to go near any island or reef for fishing or landing purposes, we always kept a safe margin of distance away, which probably accounts for our continued immunity from accident while in tortuous waters. Our anchors and cables were, however, always kept ready for use now, in case of an unsuspected current or sudden storm; but beyond that precaution, I could see little or no

> difference in the manner of our primitive navigation.
>
> ... At last we sighted the stupendous peak of Comoro mountain, which towers to nearly nine thousand feet from the little island which gives its name to the Comoro group of four. On that same day a school of medium-sized sperm whales were sighted, which appeared to be almost of a different race to those with which we had hitherto had dealings. They were exceedingly fat and lazy, moving with the greatest deliberation, and, when we rushed in among them, appeared utterly bewildered and panic-stricken, knowing not which way to flee. Like a flock of frightened sheep they huddled together, aimlessly wallowing in each other's way, while we harpooned them with the greatest ease and impunity.

Oh dear, there is quite a lot of gore after that bit. But yes, I see your point.

[Editor's note: Bullen, though undoubtedly a good writer, uses certain terms and examples of dialect that are no longer considered appropriate; please use caution in following Miss Mason's recommendation.]

Miss Mason: Now, intelligent teachers today are well aware of the dry-as-dust character of school books, so they fall back upon the oral lesson, one of whose qualities must be that it is not *bookish*.

Miss Hagan: Ah, isn't it interesting that *bookish* then becomes a derogatory term.

Miss Mason: And, to a degree, this can be successful. Living ideas can be derived only from living minds, and so it occasionally happens that a vital spark is flashed from teacher to pupil. But this occurs only when the subject is one to which the teacher has given *original* thought. In most cases the oral lesson, or the more advanced lecture for the older ones, consists of information got up by the teacher from various books, and imparted in language a little pedantic, or a little commonplace, or a little reading-made-easy in style. At the best, the teacher is not likely to have vital interest in, and, consequently, original thought upon, a wide range of subjects. So this approach often fails because of the natural limitations of teachers.

We wish to place before the child open doors to many avenues of instruction and delight, in each one of which he should find quickening thoughts. Our aim in education is to give a full life. But we cannot expect a school to be manned by a dozen master-minds, and even if it were, and the scholar were taught by each in turn, it would be much to his disadvantage. What he wants of his teacher is moral and mental discipline, sympathy and direction; and it is better, on the whole, that the training of the pupil should be undertaken by one wise teacher than that he should be passed from hand to hand for this subject and that.

Miss Hagan: What is it that we are responsible to give them?

Miss Mason: No, not quite *give* this time. We owe it to children to *initiate* an immense number of interests; "Thou hast set my feet in a large room" (Psalm 31:8) should be the glad cry of every intelligent soul; but we cannot *give* the children these interests. I know you may bring a horse to the water, but you cannot make him drink; but what I complain of is that we do *not* bring our horse to the water. We give him miserable little text-books, mere compendiums of facts, which he is to learn off, and say, and produce at an examination; or we give him various knowledge in the form of warm diluents, prepared by his teacher with perhaps some grains of living thought to the gallon. And all the time we have books, books teeming with ideas fresh from the minds of thinkers upon every subject to which we can wish to introduce children. It is rather like keeping a boat anchored close to the shore, and complaining that we cannot catch enough fish, when the waters are full of them.

Life should be all living, and not merely a tedious passing of time; not all doing or all feeling or all thinking–the strain would be too great–but, all living; that is to say, we should be in touch wherever we go, whatever we hear, whatever we see, with some manner of vital interest. We prefer that students should never say they have learned botany or conchology, geology or astronomy. The question is not,–how much does the youth *know*? when he has finished his education–but how much does he *care*? and about how many orders of things does he care? In fact, how large is the room in which he finds his feet set? and, therefore, how full is the life he has before him?

Miss Hagan: Is it not perhaps expecting too much of children to be interested in such things? Are these methods really suitable for the average student?

Miss Mason: Of course there are highly gifted and precocious children, the ones who are reading at two years of age and composing at five, the Morrises and Macaulays. But *all* children are reasonable beings. Our grandfathers and grandmothers recognized children as persons of mind and conscience like themselves, but, needing their guidance and control, as having neither knowledge nor experience. This is the note of home-life in the last generation *[Study 1]*. So soon as the baby recognized his surroundings, he found himself morally and intellectually responsible. And children have not altered. This is how we find them—with intelligence more acute, logic more keen, observing powers more alert, moral sensibilities more quick, love and faith and hope more abounding; in fact, in all points as adults are, only more so; but absolutely ignorant of the world and its belongings, of us and our ways, and, above all, of how to control and direct and manifest the infinite possibilities with which they are born.

Miss Hagan: And how do we do that?

Miss Mason: The chief aim of education is the formation of character. Character is the result not merely of the great ideas which are given to us, but of the habits which we labour to form upon those ideas. Knowing that the brain is the physical seat of habit and that conduct and character, alike, are the outcome of the habits we allow;

knowing, too, that an inspiring idea initiates a new habit of thought, and hence, a new habit of life; we perceive that the great work of education is to inspire children with vitalizing ideas as to every relation of life, every department of knowledge, every subject of thought; and to give deliberate care to the formation of those habits of the good life which are the outcome of vitalizing ideas. When we recognize both of those principles, the result is a wide range of possibilities in education, practical methods, and a definite aim. And in this great work we seek and assuredly find the co-operation of the Divine Spirit, whom we recognize, in a sense rather new to modern thought, as the supreme Educator of humankind in things that have been called secular, fully as much as in those that have been called sacred.

As to the distinguishing marks of a book for the school-room: in former times, it was sometimes thought that the bigness of a book, or the number of its volumes, showed the greatness of the writer, and swelled the virtue of the reader. But, now, big men write little books, to be used with discretion; because some of the little books are no more than abstracts, the dry bones of the subjects; but others are fresh and living. Again, we need not always insist that a book should be written by the original thinker. It sometimes happens that second-rate minds have assimilated the matter in hand, and are able to give out what is their own thought (only because they have *made* it their own) in a form more suitable for our purpose than that of the first-hand thinkers. A book may be long or short, old or new, easy or hard, written by an important person or a lesser one, and yet be the *living* book which finds its way to the mind of a young reader. The expert is not the person to choose; the children themselves are the experts in this case.

Miss Hagan: That seems to contradict something you said a few minutes ago, that the question is not what the child *likes*, as we would say they *like* sweets but *need* something more sustaining on the dinner table.

Miss Mason: In this case, the problem is that the reading of a single page by the student will elicit a verdict on the book; but that verdict is often not betrayed overtly, it is simply acted upon in the opening or closing of the door of the mind. Many excellent and admirable school-books appreciated by teachers are on the rejection list of the student; and that is why he or she takes nothing in, and gives nothing out, as we sometimes see by the poor narrations of a whole class. The distinction may be between "interests" and "relations," in the sense that interests may be fleeting, but relations are of a longer duration; and we desire that students not only find their books "interesting," but that they form enduring relationships with them.

Teachers must have it in them to distinguish between twaddle and simplicity, and between vivacity and life. For the rest they must experiment or test the experiments of others, being assured of one thing—that a book serves the ends of education only as it is *vital*.

Miss Hagan: I think I see. To use the illustration of food, a dish may be nourishing, and thought by the adults to be quite delicious, but something about its texture, perhaps, makes it disagreeable to a child who usually eat his dinner without complaint. Our first thought might be that the child is ill or upset; but if none of those things are so, we must consider the food itself.

Miss Mason: I would suggest that, in that case, the adults might do well to pay better attention, as the child might be quite right, the milk has gone sour or the cook has forgotten the salt. But it is also true that certain dishes are simply not much enjoyed by many children, we know not why.

[As on a previous occasion, the interview is ended by a knock at the door and a hurried conference with one of the college staff.]

Oh dear, I do apologize, but it appears that we have an urgent matter to settle before the last post goes out today. The secretary will give you some of our printed material and this month's copy of the *Parents' Review*, and I will also write to you on a few remaining points.

Miss Hagan: It has been such an honour to meet you, Miss Mason, and I am becoming more and more fascinated by the work of the Parents' Union. Might I also pick up an application for the House of Education?

Study 19: What Miss Hagan Took With Her

Parents' Union Prospectus

Preliminary Considerations

The Parents' Review School, an output of the Parents' Union, was, in the first place, designed to bring home-schools, taught by governesses, up to the standard of other schools. A Training College for governesses, with Practising School, etc., was established later. Children may not enter the School under six; because we think the first six years of life are wanted for physical growth and the self-education which children carry on with little ordered aid. The Parents' Review School is conducted by means of programmes of work, in five classes, sent out, term by term, to each of the home schools (and to some other schools); and the same programmes are used in the Practising School. Examination papers are set at the end of each term.

The work is arranged on the principles which will be set forth here. It consists of a wide curriculum, a considerable number of books for each child in the several classes, and, besides, a couple of hours' work daily, not with Books but with Things. Many of the pupils in the school have absorbed, in a way, the culture of their parents; but the children of uncultured parents take with equal readiness and comparable results to this sort of work, which is, I think, fitted, not only for the clever, but for the average and even the dull child.

What is Education?

The answer we accept to this question is that *Education is the Science of Relations.* We do not use this phrase in the Herbartian sense, that things or thoughts are related to each other and that teachers must be careful to pack the right things, in together, so that, having got into the pupil's brain, each may fasten on its kind, and, together, make a strong "apperception mass." What concerns us personally is the fact that we have relations with what there is in the present and with what there has been in the past, with what is above us, and about us; and that fulness of living and serviceableness depend for each of us upon how far we apprehend these relationships and how many of them we lay hold of.

Every child is heir to an enormous patrimony. The question is, what are the formalities necessary to put him in possession of that which is his?

Education Objective, not Subjective

The point of view is shifted; it is no longer *subjective* as regards the child, but *objective.* We do not talk about developing his faculties, training his moral nature, guiding his religious feelings, educating him with a view to his social standing or his future calling. We take the child as we find him, a person with many healthy affinities and embryonic attachments, and we try to give him a chance to make the largest possible number of these attachments valid. An infant comes into the world with a thousand feelers which he at once begins to fix with great energy; and out of everything about him he gets—

> That calm delight which, if I err not, surely must belong,
> To those first-born affinities that fit
> Our new existence to existing things,
> And in our dawn of being, constitute
> The bond of union between life and joy.
>
> (William Wordsworth, *The Prelude)*

He gets also when left to himself that real knowledge about each thing he comes across which establishes his relations with that thing. Our part is to remove obstructions, to give stimulus and guidance to the child who is trying to get into touch with the universe of things and thoughts.

Utilitarian Education

To educate children for any immediate end–towards commercial or manufacturing aptitude, for example–is to put a premium upon general ignorance with a view to such special aptitude. The greater includes the less, but the less does not include the greater. Excellent work of whatever kind is produced by a person of character and intelligence, and we who teach cannot do better for the nation than to prepare such persons for its uses. He who has intelligent relations with life will produce good work.

A child should be brought up to have relations of force with earth and water, should run and ride, swim and skate, lift and carry; should know texture, and work in material; should know by name, and where and how they live at any rate, the things of the earth about him, its birds and beasts and creeping things, its herbs and trees; should be in touch with the literature, art and thought of the past and the present. When he reads about the recent discoveries on Crete, for example, he should understand the excitement felt by the citizens there, as he recalls how Ulysses told Penelope about Crete with its ninety cities, and Knossos, and King Minos. He should feel that thrill *because* he has that relationship of living, pulsing thought with the past; and, if blood be thicker than water, thought is more quickening than blood.

He must have a living relationship with the present, its historic movement, its science, literature, art, social needs and aspirations. In fact, he must have a wide outlook, intimate relations all round; and force, *virtue,* must pass out of him, whether of hand, will, or sympathy, wherever he touches. This is no impossible programme. Indeed it can be pretty well filled in by the time an intelligent boy or girl has reached the age of thirteen or fourteen; for it depends, not upon *how much* is learned, but upon *how* things are learned.

Is There an "Educated Child?"

Knowledge is, no doubt, a comparative term, and the knowledge of a subject possessed by a child would be the ignorance of a student. All the same, there is such a thing as an educated child—a child who possesses a sound and wide knowledge of a number of subjects, all of which serve to interest him; such a child studies with delight.

It will be said with truth that most children do delight in school; they delight in the stimulus of school life, in the social stir of companionship; they are emulous, eager for reward and praise; they enjoy the thousand lawful interests of school life, including the attractive personality of such and such a teacher; but it seems doubtful whether the love of knowledge, in itself and for itself; is usually a powerful motive with the young scholar. The matter is important, because, of all the joyous motives of school life, the love of knowledge is the only abiding one; the only one which determines the scale, so to speak, upon which the person will hereafter live. My contention is, to repeat what has been said, that all children have a capacity for and a latent love of knowledge; and, that knowledge concerning persons and States can best be derived from books, and should be got by the children out of their own books.

Relations and Interests

I have spoken of "relations," and not of "interests," because interests may be casual, unworthy, and passing. Everyone, even the most ignorant, has interests of a sort; while to make valid any one relation, implies that knowledge has begun in, at any rate, that one direction. But the defect in our educational thought is that we have ceased to realize that knowledge is vital; and, as children and adults, we suffer from underfed minds. This intellectual inanition is, no doubt, partly due to the fact that educational theorists systematically depreciate knowledge. Such theorists are, I think, inclined to attach more importance to the working of the intellectual machinery than to the output of the product; that is, they feel it to be more important that a child should *think* than that he should *know*. My contention is rather that he cannot *know* without having *thought;* and also that he cannot think without an abundant, varied, and regular supply of the material of knowledge. We all know how the reading of a passage may stimulate in us thought, inquiry, inference, and thus get for us in the end some added knowledge.

I think there is danger in giving *too* prominent a place to education by *Things*, enormous as is its value; a certain want of atmosphere is apt to result, and a deplorable absence of a standard of comparison and of the principle of veneration. "We are the people!" seems to be the note of an education which is not largely sustained on *Books* as well as on *Things*. The depreciation of which I speak is by no means of set purpose, nor is it even realized; but the more education presents itself as a series of psychological problems, the greater will be the tendency to doctor, modify, and practically eliminate knowledge—that knowledge, which is as the air, and the food, and the exercise, the whole life of the mind of man. In giving "education" without abundant knowledge, we are as persons who should aim at physical development by giving the maximum of exercise with the minimum of food. The getting of knowledge, and the getting of *delight* in knowledge, are the ends of a child's education.

Causes of Failure

I believe that our efforts at intellectual education often fail from six causes:

(a) The oral lesson, which at its worst is very poor twaddle, and at its best is far below the ordered treatment of the same subject by an original mind in the right book. (The right books exist, old and new, in countless numbers, but very great care is necessary in the choice, as well as much experience of the rather whimsical tastes and distastes of children.)
(b) The lecture, commonly gathered from various books in rapid notes by the teacher; and issuing in hasty notes, afterwards written out, and finally crammed up by the pupils.
(c) The text-book, compressed and re-compressed from one or many big books. These handbooks are of two kinds—the frankly dry and uninteresting, which enumerate facts and details; and the easy and beguiling. I think we are safe in saying that there is *no educational value* in either sort of text-book.
(d) The debauchery of the mind which comes of exciting other desires to do the work of the inherent and fully adequate desire of knowledge.
(e) In elementary schools, the dependence upon apparatus and illustrative appliances which have a paralyzing effect on the mind.
(f) Again in elementary schools, the use of "Readers," which, however well selected, cannot have the value of consecutive works.

Subjects Covered

The first six years' work–from ages six to twelve–should and does result in the power of the pupils—

To grasp the sense of a passage of some length at a single reading: and to narrate the substance of what they have read or heard.

To spell, and express themselves in writing with ease and fair correctness.

To give an orderly and detailed account of any subject they have studied.

To describe in writing what they have seen, or heard from the newspapers.

In Arithmetic, they should have some knowledge of vulgar and decimal fractions, percentage, household accounts, etc. They should have a knowledge of Elementary Algebra, and should have done practical exercises in Geometry.

Of elementary Latin Grammar: they should read fables and easy tales, and, say, one or two books of "Caesar." They should have some power of understanding spoken French, and be able to speak a little; and to read an easy French book without a dictionary. In German, much the same as in French, but less progress.

In History, they will have gone through a rather detailed study of English, French, and Classical History.

In Geography they will have studied in detail the map of the world, and have been at one time able to fill in the landscape, industries, etc., from their studies, of each division of the map. They will have learned the elements of Physical Geography, Botany, Human Physiology, and Natural History, and will have read interesting books on some of these subjects.

They should have some knowledge of English Grammar.

They should have a considerable knowledge of Scripture History and the Bible text.

They should have learned a good deal of Scripture and of Poetry, and should have read some Literature.

In Music, they should have learned to sing on the Tonic Sol-fa method, and should know a number of English, French, and German Songs. Their knowledge of theory and their ear-training should keep pace with their powers of execution.

In Physical Activity, they should have learned Swedish Drill and various drills and calisthenic exercises.

In Drawing they should be able to represent common objects of the house and field with brush or charcoal; should be able to give rudimentary expression to ideas; and should be acquainted with the works of some artists through reproductions.

They should have skill in various handicrafts, as cardboard Sloyd, basket-making, clay-modelling, etc.

This is the degree of progress an average pupil of twelve should have made under a teacher of knowledge and ability.

Notes on Specific Subjects

Religion

For *Religion* it is, no doubt, to the Bible itself we must go, as the great storehouse of spiritual truth and moral impressions. A child might, in fact, receive a liberal education from the Bible alone, for the Book contains within itself a great literature. There was a time when "National Schools" brought up their scholars on one of the three great bodies of ancient classical literature which the Western world possesses, and which we include under the one name, Bible; and, perhaps, there has been some falling off both in national intelligence and character since the Bible has been practically deposed for the miscellaneous "Reader." It is not possible or desirable to revert to old ways in this matter; but we should see to it that children derive as much intellectual, as well as moral and religious, nutriment from books as they did when their studies ranged from the story of Joseph to the Epistles of St. Paul.

History

In *History*, boys and girls of twelve to fourteen should have a fairly intimate knowledge of English history, of contemporary French history, and of Greek and Roman history—the last, by way of biography, as perhaps nothing outside of the Bible has the educational value of Plutarch's *Lives*. They stand alone in literature as teaching that a man is part of the State, that his business is to be of service to the State, but that the value of his service depends upon his personal character.

Science

In *Science*, or rather, *Natural History*, we attach great importance to *recognition*, believing that the power to recognize and name a plant or stone or constellation involves classification and includes a good deal of knowledge. To know a plant by its gesture and habitat, its time and its way of flowering and fruiting; a bird by its flight and song and its times of coming and going; to know when, year after year, you may come upon the redstart and the pied fly-catcher, means a good deal of interested observation, and of; at any rate, the material for science.

On one afternoon in the week, the children of the Practising School go for a nature walk with their teachers. They notice for themselves, and the teacher gives a name or other information as it is asked for, and it is surprising what a range of knowledge a child of nine or ten acquires. The teachers are careful *not* to make these nature walks an opportunity for scientific instruction, as we wish the children's attention to be given to observation with very little direction. In this way they lay up that store of "common information" which Huxley considered should precede science teaching *[Study 9]*; and, what is much more important, they learn to know and delight in natural objects as in the familiar faces of friends. The children keep a dated record of what they see in their nature note-books, which are left to their own management and are not corrected. These note-books are a source of pride and joy, and are freely illustrated by drawings (brushwork) of twig, flower, insect, etc. The knowledge necessary for these records is not given in the way of teaching.

We supplement the nature walk by occasional object-lessons, as, on the hairs of plants, on diversity of wings, on the sorts of matters taken up in Professor Miall's capital books; but our dependence is on *books* as an adjunct to the out-of-door work.

Picture Talks

We attach a good deal of value to what we call *picture talks*. A reproduction of a suitable picture, by Millet, for example, is put into the students' hands, and they study it by themselves. Then, children of from six to nine describe the picture, giving all the details and showing by a few lines on the blackboard where is such a tree or such a house; judging if they can the time of day; discovering the story if there be one. The older children add to this some study of the lines of composition, light and shade, the particular style of the master; and reproduce from memory certain details.

The object of these lessons is that students should learn how to appreciate rather than how to produce.

Some Benefits of this Approach

1. The cost of the books per pupil for the six years–from six to twelve–does not average more than one pound a year. A scheme of work for elementary schools might be arranged at a much less annual cost for books.

2. Two and a half, for Class I., to three and a half hours a day, for Class III., is ample time for this book education.

3. Much writing is unnecessary, because the pupils have the matter in their books and know where to find it.

4. Classes II. and III. are able to occupy themselves in study with pleasure and profit.

5. Teachers are relieved of the drudgery of many corrections.

6. The pupils have the afternoons for handicrafts, nature-work, walks, games, etc.

7. The evenings are free, whether at school or at home, for reading aloud, choral singing, hobbies, etc.

8. The pupils get many intelligent interests, beget hobbies, and have leisure for them.

9. There is no distressing cramming for the term's examination. The pupils know their work, and find it easy to answer questions set to find out what they know, rather than what they do not know.

10. Children of any age, however taught hitherto, take up this sort of work with avidity.

11. Boys and girls taught in this way take up ordinary school work, preparation for examinations, etc., with intelligence, zeal, and success.

Should the reader consider that the children in question prove their right of entry to several fields of knowledge, that they show a distinct appetite for such knowledge, that thought and power of mind develop upon the books we read, as they do not and cannot upon the lectures we hear; should he indeed be convinced of the truth of what I have advanced, I think he will see that, not an educational reform here and there, but an entire ***Educational Revolution*** is before us, to which every one of us is bound to put his hand.

Study 20: Using Books (Letters from Miss Mason to Miss Hagan)

May 15, 1904

Dear Miss Hagan,

It was indeed a pleasure to meet you, and I hope that the readers of your father's newspaper will gain some new and valuable ideas after reading your story. I am also happy to hear of your personal interest in studying our methods.

As I recall, we had discussed the choosing of the "right" books [*Study 18*]; but the right *use* of them is another matter. This is the challenge: that, having found the right book, the teacher must give the book the lead and be content to take second place. The lecture *must be subordinated to the book*. So then, what is the business of the teacher? To put her class in the right attitude towards that book, by a word or two of her own interest in the matter contained, and of her own delight in the manner of the author. The children must enjoy the book. The ideas it holds must each make that sudden, delightful impact upon their minds, must cause that intellectual stir, which mark the inception of an idea. The teacher's part in this regard is to see and feel for himself, and then to rouse his pupils by an appreciative look or word; but to beware how he deadens the impression by a flood of talk. Intellectual sympathy is very stimulating; but we have all been in the case of the little girl who said, "Mother, I think I could understand if you did not explain *quite* so much." A teacher said of her pupil, "I find it so hard to tell whether she has really grasped a thing or whether she has only got the mechanical hang of it." It is only the "mechanical hang" that is apt to arrive after such a shower of explanation.

Labour, as we discussed, prepares the way for assimilation, that mental process which converts information into knowledge; and the effort of taking in the sequence of thought of his author is worth to the child a great deal of oral teaching. (Do teachers not realize the paralyzing and stupefying effect that a flood of talk has upon the mind?) The inspired talk of an orator no doubt wakens a response and is listened to with tense attention; but few of us claim to be inspired, and we are sometimes aware of the difficulty of holding the attention of a class. We blame ourselves, whereas the blame lies in the instrument we employ—the more or less diluted oral lesson or lecture, in place of the living and arresting book. Of course we cannot do without the oral lesson—to introduce, to illustrate, to amplify, to sum up. But my stipulation is that oral lessons should be few and far between.

And what about educational appliances? "Appliance" can be both a tool intended for a specific purpose, and something fitted by a doctor or a dentist for correction. Both meanings amplify our reasons for being cautious in the use of appliances: first, that they are often limited in uses, and not a good investment of funds; and, second, that such things may carry a *surgical* flavour—that is, they are brought in to correct a thing that never was out of alignment. But, even more than that, like too many oral lessons, we find that they tend to *paralyze* the mental vigour of children.

I have not specified exactly what sort of appliances I am criticizing, and indeed we do allow the microscope, telescope, magic lantern pictures, etc. But here is an example of what we do *not* need: I once heard a schoolmaster, who had a school in a shipbuilding town, say that he had demanded and got from his committee a complete sectional model of a man-of-war. Such a model would be of use to his boys when they begin to work in the Yards; but during their school years I believe the effect would be stultifying, because the mind is not able to conceive with an elaborate model as basis.

I recently visited M. Bloch's admirable "Peace and War" show at Lucerne. Torpedoes were very fully illustrated by models, sectional diagrams, and what not, but I was not enlightened. I asked my neighbour at dinner to explain the principle; he took up his spectacle case as an illustration, and after a few sentences my intelligence had grasped what was distinctive in a torpedo. This gentleman turned out to have been in the War Office and to have had much concern with torpedoes. The power in the teacher of illustrating by inkpot and ruler or any object at hand, or by a few lines on the blackboard, appears to me to be of more use than the most elaborate equipment of models and diagrams; these things stale on the senses and produce a torpor of thought the moment they are presented.

Yours sincerely…

May 21, 1904

Dear Miss Hagan,

Is "getting ideas out of them" all we must do with books? By no means. "In all labour there is profit" (Prov. 14:23), or at any rate in *some* labour; and the labour of *thought* is what his book must induce in the child. He must generalize, classify, infer, judge, visualize, discriminate, labour in one way or another, with that capable mind of his, until the substance of his book is assimilated or rejected, according as he shall determine; for the determination rests with him and not with his teacher.

Now I do not recall that we spoke much of *narration*, and that was certainly an oversight on my part. The simplest way of dealing with a paragraph or a chapter is to require the child to narrate its contents after a single attentive reading,—one reading, however slow, should be made a condition; for we (as adults) are all too apt to make sure we shall have another opportunity of finding out something to which we did not pay close enough attention. There is the weekly review if we fail to get a clear grasp of the news of the day; and, if we fail a second time, there is a monthly review, or the "annual": in fact, many of us let present-day history pass by us with easy minds, feeling sure that, in the end, we shall be *compelled* to see the bearings of events. This is a bad habit to get into; and we should do well to save our children by not giving them the expectation of second and third (and tenth) opportunities to do that which should have been done at first.

There is much difference between intelligent reading, which the pupil should do in silence, and a mere parrot-like cramming up of contents; and it is not a bad test of education to be able to give the points of a description, the sequence of a series of incidents, the links in a chain of argument, correctly, after a single careful reading. This is a power which a barrister, a publisher, a scholar, labours to acquire, as I am sure you have found yourself in your newspaper work; and it is a power which children can acquire with great ease, and once acquired, the gulf is bridged which divides the reading from the non-reading community.

But oral narration is only one way to use books: others are to enumerate the statements in a given paragraph or chapter; to analyze a chapter, to divide it into paragraphs under proper headings, to tabulate and classify series; to trace cause to consequence and consequence to cause; to discern character and perceive how character and circumstance interact; to get lessons of life and conduct, or the living knowledge which makes for science, out of books. All this is possible for school boys and girls, and *until* they have begun to use books for themselves in such ways, they can hardly be said to have begun their education.

So, you might wonder, what then is the "mother hen" teacher doing while the chicks are scratching (if you recall my nursery rhyme)? The teacher's part is, in the first place, to see what is to be done, to look over the work of the day in advance and see what mental discipline, as well as what vital knowledge, this and that lesson afford; and then to set questions and tasks such as shall give full scope to his pupils' mental activity.

Let marginal notes be freely made (as neatly and beautifully as may be, for books should be handled with reverence). Let numbers, letters, underlining be used to help the eye and to save the needless drudgery of writing abstracts. Let the pupil write for himself half a dozen questions which cover the passage studied; he need not write the answers if he be taught that "the mind can know nothing but what it can produce in the form of an answer to a question put by the mind to itself."

Yours sincerely…

May 27, 1904

Dear Miss Hagan,

No, unfortunately, I cannot remember the exact source of that quotation with which I ended my last letter. I once heard it from an old philosopher, but I do not know where he found it. But nevertheless it is useful, don't you think?

Yes, that was quite the long list of disciplinary devices, and they all have their uses; but we must be careful that our disciplinary devices, and our mechanical devices to secure and tabulate the substance of knowledge, do not come between the children and that which is the *soul* of the book, the living thought it contains. Science is doing so much for us in these days, nature is drawing so close to us, art is unfolding so much meaning to us, the world is becoming so rich for us, that we are a little in danger of neglecting the art of deriving sustenance from books. Let us not in such wise impoverish our lives and the lives of our children; for, to quote the golden words of Milton:

> Books are not absolutely dead things, but do contain a potency of life in them to be as active as that soul was, whose progeny they are; nay, they do preserve, as in a vial, the purest efficacy and extraction of that living intellect that bred them. As good almost kill a man, as kill a good book; who kills a man kills a good reasonable creature, God's image; but he who destroys a good book, kills reason itself—kills the image of God, as it were, in the eye.

Responding to your question about education by *Things* (rather than books), yes, we do put a great value on such teaching, as it builds the important *affinities* with the earth and all that is in it, not to mention helping to strengthen our bodies and make us more useful and serviceable to others. But, at the present time (I am happy to say), education by *Things* seems to be everywhere, and such activities as handicrafts are seen to make for education as truly as do geography and Latin. The teaching of Science is also receiving enormous attention. What everyone knows it is unnecessary to repeat; so I have been attempting to bring things more into balance, as it were, with talk about the more-and-more neglected art of education by *Books*.

Still, I thought you might be interested in these notes from a Picture Talk given to a class of thirteen-year-olds.

OBJECTS.

1. To give the girls some idea of composition, based on the work of the artist Jean-François Millet.
2. To inspire them with a desire to study the works of other artists, with a similar object in view.
3. To help them with their original illustrations, by giving them ideas, carried out in Millet's work, as to simplicity of treatment, breadth of tone, and use of lines.

MATERIALS NEEDED.

Paint-boxes, brushes, pencils, etc. Prints of some of Millet's pictures.

LESSON.

Step 1. Introduce the subject by talking with the students about their original illustrations. Tell them how our great artists have drawn ideas and inspiration from the work of other artists; have studied their pictures, copied them, and tried to get at the spirit of them. Tell them that today we are going to study some of the pictures of the great French artist Jean-François Millet.

Step 2. Tell the students a little about the life of Millet (giving them one or two pictures to look at meanwhile); give only a brief sketch, so that they will feel that he is not a stranger to them. Talk to them a little about his childhood, how he worked in the fields; how he had two great "books"—the Book of Nature and the Bible, from which he drew much inspiration; how later on he went to Paris and studied the pictures of great artists, Michael Angelo among them.

Step 3. Show the pictures to the students, let them look well at them, and then draw from them their ideas as to the beauty and simplicity of the composition; call attention to the breadth of tone, and the dignity of the lines. Help them, sketching when necessary. to reduce a picture to its most simple form; half-closing their eyes to shut out detail, help them to get an idea of the masses of tone, etc.

Step 4. Let the children reproduce a detail of one of the pictures, working in watercolour with monochrome and making their washes simple and flat, reducing the tones to two or three.

Step 5. (Optional) Encourage the students to look equally carefully at the style, details, etc. in other places, whether that is in one of Caldecott's Picture Books, or in the paintings of some other artist.

You also had some questions about the use of the Bible in schools and family life, besides in the Church itself. I firmly believe that the Bible is a great storehouse of moral impressions—and the Bible itself, not a compendium of its teaching. Have you read Thomas De Quincey on this subject, in his *Autobiographic Sketches*?

> It had happened, that among our vast nursery collection of books was the Bible, illustrated with many pictures. And in long dark evenings, as my three sisters with myself sat by the firelight round the guard of our nursery, no book was so much in request amongst us.

De Quincey is here recalling the sudden death of his sister Elizabeth. He was told that she had died, and crept into her room, wanting to see her once more; but the bed had been moved, and all he could see at first was an open window:

> through which the sun of midsummer, at midday, was showering down torrents of splendor. The weather was dry, the sky was cloudless, the blue depths seemed the express types of infinity; and it was not possible for eye to behold, or for heart to conceive, any symbols more pathetic of life and the glory of life.

He explains why, then and afterwards, he made such personal connections between summer and sunshine, mortality and death; that through his nurse's comments on the Bible stories, the impression he had gotten of Palestine, and Jerusalem in particular, was that it seemed to be a place of everlasting summer, but a summer particularly connected with death (because of the death of Christ).

> There [in Jerusalem] it was, indeed, that the human had risen on wings from the grave; but, for that reason, there also it was that the divine had been swallowed up by the abyss; the lesser star could not rise before the greater should submit to eclipse. Summer, therefore, had connected itself with death, not merely as a mode of antagonism, but also as a phenomenon brought into intricate relations with death by scriptural scenery and events.

Now obviously De Quincey was a more than usually perceptive and sensitive child, and you may wonder why I am quoting this story at such length. My first point is that, indeed, there is some value in reading the Bible to young children; but also, if we put it in context, we see the possibility of a deeper sense of life (and death) given through those early impressions, and then the gift of that understanding when death indeed became real.

Clearly this is one of the places where, if we were wise enough, we would draw back from tampering or commenting on the stories as much as we often do. But at the same time, we dare not deny our children the opportunity to hear them, to know them deeply, and to become aware of a sense of eternity, given with reverence, when "the wind bloweth where it listeth" (John 3:8).

Yours sincerely…

June 1, 2004

Dear Miss Hagan,

You ask why it is easier for our teachers to deal in a more "direct fashion" with knowledge? It is because we are not embarrassed by the necessity of cultivating faculties; for working purposes the so-called faculties are sufficiently described as *mind*; and the normal mind is, we find, as able to deal with knowledge as are the normal digestive organs with food. As there are gymnastics for the body, so for the mind there are certain subjects whose use is chiefly disciplinary, and of these we avail ourselves.

Again, as our various organs labour without our consciousness in the assimilation food, so judgment, imagination, and what not, deal their own accord with knowledge, that it may be *incorporated*. As the digestive organs are incited by appetite, so children come into the world with a few inherent desires, some with more, some less, to incite them to their proper activities. These are, roughly speaking, the desire for power, for praise, for wealth, for distinction, for society, and for *knowledge*.

It seems to me that education which appeals to the desire for wealth (marks, prizes, scholarships, or the like), or to the desire of excelling (as in the taking of places, etc.), or to any other of the natural desires, *except that for knowledge*, destroys the balance of character; and, what is even more fatal, destroys by inanition that desire for and delight in knowledge which is meant for our joy and enrichment through the whole of life. "A desire for knowledge," says Dr. Johnson, "is the natural feeling of mankind, and every human being whose mind is not debauched will be willing to give all that he has to get knowledge." Is it possible that what has been called "mark-hunger" is a debauchery of the mind? The undebauched mind takes knowledge with avidity; and we find their studies are so interesting to children that they need no other stimulus.

One other practical reason that our teachers say these practices are "easier" is that the use of books makes for short hours. No book-work or writing, no preparation or report, is done in the Parents' Review school, except between the hours of 9:00 and 11:30 for the lowest class, to 9:00 and 1:00 for the highest, with half an hour's interval for drill, etc. From one to two hours, according to age and class, are given in the afternoons to handicrafts, field-work, drawing, etc.; and the evenings are free, so that the children have leisure for hobbies, family reading, and the like. We are able to get through a greater variety of subjects, and through more work in each subject, in a shorter time than is usually allowed, because children taught in this way get the habit of close attention and are carried on by steady interest.

We are often asked how we approach the "disciplinary" subjects of instruction, perhaps those that are less immediately appealing to young minds, and those which require a continuous building up of new rules, like stepping stones across a river from which, if one is out of place, we may find ourselves in deep water. Well, first of all we must choose which of those subjects will be in the curriculum at all. Having cleared our minds as to the end we have in view, we ask ourselves— "Is there any fruitful idea underlying this or that study that the children are engaged in?" We divest ourselves of the notion that to develop the faculties is the chief thing; and a "subject" which does not rise out of some great thought of life we usually reject as not nourishing, not fruitful; while we retain those studies which give exercise in habits of clear and orderly thinking. Mathematics, grammar, logic, etc., are not purely disciplinary; they do develop, if you will allow the expression, intellectual *muscle*. We by no means reject the familiar staples of education in the school sense, but we prize them even more for the record of intellectual habits they leave in the brain tissue.

And as for how these subjects may be best taught? Give children a wide range of subjects, with the end in view of establishing in each case some one or more of the relations I have indicated. Let them learn from first-hand sources of information—really good books, the best going, on the subject they are engaged upon. Let them get at the books themselves, and do not let them be flooded with talk from the lips of their teacher. The teacher's business is to indicate, stimulate, direct and constrain to the acquirement of knowledge, but by no means to be the fountain-head and source of all knowledge in his or her own person. Children must be allowed to ruminate: to contemplate, or (more literally) to graze for their own nourishment, and chew it over as needed. They must be left alone with their own thoughts, and they will ask for help if they want it.

But we may not choose or reject subjects at our own whim. You will see at a glance, with this Captain Idea of establishing relationships as a guide, the unwisdom of choosing or rejecting this or that subject, as being more or less useful or necessary in view of a child's future. We decide, for example, that Tommy, who is eight, need not waste his time over the Latin Grammar. We intend him for commercial or scientific pursuits, so what good will it be to him? But we do not know how much we are shutting out from Tommy's range of thought *besides* Latin grammar. He has to translate, for example,– "*Pueri formosos equos vident*" (The boys see the beautiful horses), from *A Child's First Latin Book*). He is a ruminant animal (as above), and has been told something about that strong Roman people whose speech is now brought before him. How their boys catch hold of him! How he gloats over their horses! The Latin grammar is not mere words to Tommy, or rather Tommy knows, as we have forgotten, that the epithet *mere* is the very last to apply to words.

Of course it is only now and then that a notion catches the small boy; but when it does catch, it works wonders, and does more for his education than years of grind.

I think you will be able to discern much of this through the prospectus you received, but again there is much to be gained by direct teaching and practical experience. If you are indeed planning on joining our next class, please let Miss Kitching know soon, as she will need to send you the particulars.

Yours sincerely,

Charlotte M. Mason

Notes for a New Era

The Heart Is a Lonely Affinity-Hunter

Some Christians are uncomfortable with the idea of "Jesus in our hearts." I know one Sunday school teacher who told her class, "The heart is just a pump. Maybe we should ask Jesus to come into our brains instead."

But have you ever heard of the intracardiac nervous system? It's been known for a couple of decades that the heart is controlled not only by the brain, but by a more "local" system of neurons—40,000 of them, in fact. In popular language, we're now told that "the heart has its own 'brain,'" and that biologists have more recently been able to draw a detailed 3-D map of the "little brain."

What does that mean? Well, to begin with, that the heart, in some sense, feels its own pain—physiological, but perhaps also emotional. Perhaps those who first described "heartache" were closer to the truth than they knew.

And, for those who have marvelled at the complexity and plasticity of the brain itself, this seems to give us one more confirmation that we do not think, or learn, or feel, in purely mechanical ways. We may ask *why* a particular poem touches us spiritually, but perhaps we should also ask *where.*

Miss Mason wrote that

> As the digestive organs are incited by appetite, so children come into the world with a few inherent desires, some with more, some less, to incite them to their proper activities. These are, roughly speaking, the desire for power, for praise, for wealth, for distinction, for society, and for knowledge.

And now we can ask—are those desires purely in the brain (and we've discovered that we can't say exactly which part of the brain)? Or do they come also from the heart?

Perhaps the scientists will, at long last, agree with the poets.

The Question of Competition

> It seems to me that education which appeals to the desire for wealth (marks, prizes, scholarships, or the like), or to the desire of excelling (as in the taking of places, etc.), or to any other of the natural desires, except that for knowledge, destroys the balance of character; and, what is even more fatal, destroys by inanition that desire for and delight in knowledge which is meant for our joy and enrichment through the whole of life.

In twenty-first century culture, for a number of deeply-felt reasons, we seem to be divided on the question of merit-based rewards, and also punishments. For instance, it is rare that a child is bluntly said to have failed in school. And there have been many attempts, over the years, to promote co-operative versions of games, where the fun is simply in the playing, and "everybody wins." Such initiatives have to be applauded for their attempts to promote kindness and acceptance of others. At the same time, we as a culture adore success and status; we love to know that "our team" has won the trophy. And we hear of parents who push their children to excel in academics or sports or the arts, to the unhappiness of all concerned.

Further, we may criticize some of this "coddling" which now takes place in schools, saying that the real world (of work and power and so on) is not like that at all. Which workers will get promoted? We hope it's the ones who do the best work (although sometimes it's the proverbial boss's nephew, and that's also the "real world").

Is Miss Mason saying that those who show the greatest talent or diligence should not get their due reward? Is she actually criticizing all practice of prizes and scholarships? (Should we play down our personal talents so as not to make other people feel inferior?) Interestingly, the Parents' Union, from time to time, offered both (such as the Rooper Memorial Scholarship), so the answer would seem to be "no." For instance, the nature notebooks of the student teachers were submitted to an outside examiner, and his comments about each book were printed in the *Parents' Review*. The notebooks were also classed in something like the "A" group and the "B" group, as were certain other exam results, so there was certainly no shirking the idea that superior work deserved higher praise.

However, what seems to be discussed in the passage above is the motivation behind our desire to succeed. Miss Mason describes the "cult" of physical perfection, pointing out the difference between desiring to be strong or healthy or even beautiful for one's own sake, vs. keeping one's body fit for the purpose of service. In another place, she talks about those who aim for moral perfection, but for the affirmation of their own egos. This would seem to be a similar problem, in that, ultimately, if you do a great job at something (if things are fair, though they sometimes aren't), you know that you might get a promotion. Or a scholarship, a medal, a Nobel Prize, or a sticky star.

And then again, you might not.

And that's the point.

How do we communicate that to children? How do we encourage them to aim for excellence, and acknowledge their successes (or oh-so-close-to-successes), without obsessing over external rewards? It's a tough one. Perhaps literature can help, including biographies. And the reading of verses like Romans 12:15, "Rejoice with those who rejoice, mourn with those who mourn," or Matthew 20:16, "The last shall be first, and the first last." None of that takes away the disappointment when an honest effort still isn't enough; but it can help us to keep on trying.

With Inkpot and Ruler

> The power in the teacher of illustrating by inkpot and ruler or any object at hand, or by a few lines on the blackboard, appears to me to be of more use than the most elaborate equipment of models and diagrams; these things stale on the senses and produce a torpor of thought the moment they are presented.

This amplifies the sixth principle of education, that "we do not mean that a child should be isolated in what may be called a 'child-environment' especially adapted and prepared…It stultifies a child to bring down his world to the child's level."

Our friend Wendi has often asked, "What do you have in your hand?" What is available to you, what is most cost-effective (or free), what is most flexible and versatile, and what meets the actual needs of the moment? Do children need plastic climbing equipment if their home has nearby hills and trees? I have already mentioned Mary Pride's "less-clutter" approach to lesson planning: try a simple approach first before assuming that a complicated one must be superior. And, in fact, Miss Mason seems to be saying that a complicated, detailed explanation or model may be *less* effective; and more limited.

Here is your challenge (pick one that seems most appropriate):

1. Cook or bake something using a bare-bones recipe, the kind that people used to dictate orally: "water up to the second scratch in the kettle," "butter the size of a walnut," and so on. Or hide the measuring cups and spoons, and just estimate the amounts.

2. Plan a lesson that teaches a new concept, say in math or science. Do not use any commercial manipulatives, and try to avoid using ready-made diagrams or photographs (just this time). How else can you demonstrate the idea?

3. Imagine that there is something you yourself want to learn: crocheting, small engine repair, tuning a guitar, or something not as hands-on, like the history of education. List your options (formal class, online videos, how-to books, knowledgeable friend, etc.). Try one or two of the different methods, and watch how the teacher or author communicates: simple and clear, or long and complicated? Fancy tools, or the basics? Which one do you find most effective?

Part Five: In Which the Student Teachers Compare Notes

For the last twelve years we have tried the plan of bringing children up on *Books* and *Things*, and, on the whole, the results are pleasing. The *average* child studies with "delight." We do not say he will remember all he knows, but, to use a phrase of Jane Austen's, he will have had his "imagination warmed" in many regions of knowledge. (*School Education*, p. 243)

The Children's Magna Carta.—My plea is, and I think I have justified it by experience, that many doors shall be opened to boys and girls until they are at least twelve or fourteen, and always the doors of *good* houses... that they shall be introduced to no subject whatever through compendiums, abstracts, or selections; that the young people shall learn what history is, what literature is, what life is, from the living books of those who know. I know it can be done, because it is being done on a considerable scale.

If conviction has indeed reached us, the Magna Carta of children's intellectual liberty is before us. The need is immediate, the means are evident. (*School Education*, p. 247)

Study 21: The Primary Years

We join the junior class again as they chat in their common room.

Miss Glass: When you teach the Form I class in the Practising School, don't you notice a great deal of difference between what the six-year-olds can do, compared with the oldest who have already turned nine and should be moving into the next form?

Miss Capehart: Yes, there is a great development during those years, and you see it in their narrations. But it is good, in a way, to have the younger ones working with those just a bit older; I think it keeps them challenged.

Miss Breckenridge: And sometimes the younger children make observations that are just as sharp as those of the older ones; they may not be as fluent in expressing it, especially in writing, but they do see things just as well, and they listen as carefully; perhaps not for quite as long, though.

Miss Bruce: I took the Form I class on a nature walk, and as preparation for the coming examinations, I divided them into teams by age (because that gave us even numbers), and asked each team to gather three sorts of tree leaf-buds and two sorts of catkin, and afterwards tell me all they could about them.

Miss White: Did you save their responses?

Miss Bruce: Yes, and this is what I got from the six-year-olds:

(1) The chestnut bud is brown and sticky, it is a sort of cotton-woolly [*sic*] with the leaves inside. It splits open and sends out two leaves, and the leaves split open.

(2) The oak twig bas always a lot of buds on the top, and one bud always dies. Where the bud starts there is a little bit of knot-wood. The oak-bud is very tiny.

(3) The lime bud has a green side and a red side, and then it bursts open and several little leaves come out and all the little things that shut up the leaves die away.

(4) Golden catkins and silver "pussy palms" of a willow tree. The golden catkins have stamens with all the pollen on them. They grow upwards, and two never grow opposite to each other. The silver pussy palms have seed boxes, with a little tube growing out, and a little sticky knob on the top. The bees rub the pollen off their backs on to the sticky knob.

Miss Glass: How did the nine-year-olds do?

Miss Bruce: These narrations might have been better done in language skills, but all the nine-year-olds in the class this year came to us from another school, and are slightly behind what we might expect. They did find a lot of different twigs, though!

(1) Beech Twig. —It has rather a woody stalk, and it is a very light grey-browny stalk, and it is very thin, and the little branches that grow out are light brown and it is thicker where the buds are and it is a lighter brown up at the top than it is at the bottom, and the buds are a light reddy-brown and very pointed, and they are scaly. The bark is rather rough and there is a lot of little kind of brown spots on it.

(2) Lime Twig.—It is called Ruby-budded Lime because the buds are red, and they are fat rather, and they have got some green in as well, and they come rather to a point at the top, they grow alternately and the little stalk that they grow out of is reddy-green, and the top part of the stalk is green, and it is woody, and it is rough, and it is a reddy-green at the bottom. Where the buds come out it is swelled out, the bark has come off and it has left it white and woody. At the top of one of the stalks the bud has come off.

(3) Sycamore Twig. —Well, the back is very woody, and it is a brown stalk and it is rough and there is a little weeny bud growing out of the side, and the buds grow out two and two, and there. are a lot of little buds.

(4) Willow. —Well, the stalk is a dark brown, and is very smooth and it will bend very easily, and the buds when they first come on the stalk are little brown ones, and then a silvery-green comes out and there is a scale at the bottom, and then they get greyer and bigger with little green leaves at the bottom, and then it comes yellow, and there is a lot of pollen on it. If you touch it the pollen comes on your finger.

(5) Hazel. —Well, the stalk is a dark brown, something the colour of the willow, and it bends easily, and the buds are green and there is little scales, and then the catkins come and they grow very long, and there is a lot of little flowers in one, and there is pollen in that, and the stalk is rather rough, and there are some big buds at the top just bursting, and the leaves are coming out, and the buds are very soft and glossy, and the scales are at the bottom.

Miss White: I think those were quite well done for any third-graders.

Miss Laurio: Third-graders?

Miss White: Sorry, I keep having to mentally translate my Canadian school terms into British ones. I meant those in their last year of the first form. Miss Bruce, I have been working with the older students, so I'm not as familiar yet with the programme for the little ones. How long do they work each morning?

Miss Bruce: Two and a half hours, but half an hour of that is spent in drill and games. They are reading about sixteen books this term, for the thirteen different subjects of study; and the eight- and nine-year-olds have a few more books and subjects.

They are learning both printing and cursive writing, are learning to read, and there is a great deal of oral work for the other subjects, including French. There is a lot of time spent on music and recitation, and they also do brush-drawing and handicrafts.

Miss Capehart: What about arithmetic?

Miss Bruce: All the Form I's are using a little book called *The A.B.C. of Arithmetic*, but we have had to divide them into beginners and advanced, with the advanced group working on a later chapter. They use dominoes, beans and so on to help them answer the questions, especially the word problems, such as "If 100 soldiers march in rows of four, how many rows are there?" and "If walnuts are nine shillings per hundred, how much for 50 walnuts?" One problem with this book is that many of the questions refer to "staves and cubes," and Miss Mason prefers us to say "tens and units." I think they are considering some other, newer book, but for now we still have *The A.B.C.*

Their Bible lessons are read from the Bible; tales, natural history, and geography are taught from the various books, and these are helped by the children's own observations. Our plan in each of these subjects is to read them the passage for the lesson (a good long passage), talk about it a little, avoiding much explanation, and then let them narrate what has been read. (The older ones are able to do some of their own reading.) This they do very well, and they are often happy in catching the style as well as the words of the author.

Miss Breckenridge: When I assisted with the younger children, I was struck by the correctness and copiousness of the language used, especially in their examinations.

Miss Laurio: Young children often surprise us by their free and correct use of "dictionary words." Miss Bruce and I have noticed the verve with which the children tell the tale, the orderly sequence of events, the correctness and fulness of detail, the accuracy of names. These things are natural to children—until they are schooled out of them. Here is one example from our class:

Q. Tell a fairy story.
B. (aged 6 3/4): —

When Ulysses was coming back from Troy he passed the Sirens. He could hear them, but he couldn't get to them, because he was bound.

> He wanted to get to them so as he could listen to them a long time, because a lot of people had come and listened to them, and they found it so beautiful that they wanted to stay there, and they stayed till they died. His companions couldn't hear them because they stopped up their ears with wax and cotton-wool. And this was the song they sang:—
>
> "Hither, come hither and hearken awhile,
> Odysseus far-famed king,
> No sailor has ever passed this way
> But has paused to hear us sing.
> Our song is sweeter than honey,
> And he that hears it knows
> What he never learnt from another,
> And his joy before he goes.
>
> "We know what the heroes bore at Troy
> In the ten long years of strife,
> We know what happened in all the world,
> And the secret things of life."
>
> And then they rowed on till at last the song faded away, and they rowed on and on for a long time, and then when they could not hear them nor see them, the wax was taken out of their ears, and then they unbound Ulysses.

Miss White: How did a six-year-old remember that song so well?

Miss Laurio: We found that version in a song book, and the children learned it along with their lesson. So perhaps it is not a perfect example of children hearing the story once and remembering it, but still I think it was well done.

Miss Bruce: One of the girls who is almost eight gave us this response to the question "What have you (yourself) noticed about a spider?"

> We have found out the name of one spider, and often have seen spiders under the microscope—they were all very hairy. We have often noticed a lot of spiders running about the ground—quantities [of them]. Last term we saw a spider's web up in the corner of the window with a spider sucking out the juice of a fly; and we have often touched a web to try and make the spider come out, and we never could, because she saw it wasn't a fly, before she came out. I saw the claw of a spider under the microscope, with its little teeth; we saw her spinnerets and her great eyes. There were the two big eyes in one row, four little ones in the next row, and two little ones in the next row.
>
> We have often found eggs of the spiders; we have some now that we

have got in a little box, and we want to hatch them out, so we have put them on the mantelpiece to force them.

Once we saw a spider on a leaf, and we tried to catch it, but we couldn't; he immediately let himself down on to the ground with a thread. We saw the circulation in the leg of another spider under the microscope; it looked like a little line going up and down.

Miss Glass: Now that is a child who will never forget the word "circulation." Or "spinneret."

Study 22: The Junior Years

Miss White: Miss Breckenridge, are you finding much difference between the Form I and the Form II classes? The second form are the children from nine to twelve, correct?

Miss Breckenridge: Generally, yes, although they are occasionally over twelve. They have twenty-one subjects, with the addition of Latin and German, and about twenty-five books are used. They work from 9:00 to 12:00 each day, half an hour with half an hour's interval for games and drill. In music they continue Mrs. Curwen's Child Pianist method, and Tonic Sol-fa, and learn French and English songs.

One of the biggest changes is that they do more writing, though not everything. For their examinations they may write the answers themselves, or dictate them, or some of each according to their age.

Miss Laurio: Are they doing spelling lessons?

Miss Breckenridge: Most of the students can spell reasonably well, if we go by their general success at dictation; to quote Miss Mason, "the habit of reading teaches spelling."

Miss Laurio: What are they doing in History?

Miss Breckenridge: Mr. Arnold-Forster's book is extremely popular with the students, even though it is about 800 pages long; they call it a "manly" treatment of English History, and in no case is there any writing down to them. Mrs. Creighton's *First History of France* is also a favourite, though I should have thought there was hardly enough detail to make it so. Also, they take up one of Plutarch's *Lives* each term, as they also do in Form III. The *Lives* are read to the children almost without comment, but with (ahem) necessary omissions.

The books they are reading for Natural History are also on a more serious level now, and give more scientific information, even if they have titles like *The Fairy-Land of Science*. And of course they are joining in the out-of-door nature-study, as that continues to lay the foundation for science. This term they are to notice all they can about twenty wild-flowers, and to record and describe in their nature notebooks. To help them with that, they have a little book also by Arabella Buckley, *Plant Life in Field and Garden*. It is written in a simple style that encourages them to get out their magnifying glasses and look deeper.

Miss Glass: What are they doing in the *Fairy-Land* book this term?

Miss Breckenridge: Just the chapter "Bees in the Hive"; but they have quite a bit of other reading this term in Holden's *The Sciences*: a whole section on chemistry, and then another one on meteorology: clouds, raindrops, winds, storms.

Miss Capehart: Sounds like the weather report for the Lake District, all right.

Miss Breckenridge: Here's a response from the Bees chapter, dictated by a ten-year-old.

> Q. How many kinds of bees are there in a hive? What work does each do? Tell how they build the comb.
>
> F. Three kinds. The drones or males, the workers or females, and the queen bee. The drone is fat, the queen is long and thin, the workers are small and slim. The queen bee lays the eggs, the worker bee brings the honey in and makes the cell, and the drones wait to be fed. On a summer's day you see something hanging on a tree like a plum pudding, this is a swarm of bees. You will soon see someone come up with a hive, turn it upside down, shake the bough gently, and they will fall in. They will put some clean calico quickly over the bottom of the hive, and turn it back over on a bench. The bees first close up every little hole in the hive with wax, then they hang on to the roof, clinging on to one another by their legs. Then one comes away and scrapes some wax from under its body, and bites it in its mouth until it is pulled out like ribbon, this she plasters on the roof of the hive, then she flies out to get honey, and comes home to digest it, hanging from the roof, and in 24 hours this digested honey turns to wax, then she goes through the same process again. Next, the nursing bees come and poke their heads into this wax, bite the wax away (20 bees do this before one hole is ready to make a cell). Other bees are working on the other side at the same time. Each cell is made six-sided, so as to take up the least wax and the smallest space. When the cells are made the bees come in with honey in their honey-bag or first stomach; they can easily pass the honey back though their mouths into the cells. It takes many bees to fill one cell, so they are hard at work.

Miss Bruce: I should imagine so! And for handicrafts and such?

Miss Breckenridge: Much the same as Form I: cardboard Sloyd, clay modelling, needlework, gardening, etc. But these activities have to wait for the afternoons or after teatime, as the students' time in the morning is taken up with book work, arithmetic, languages and so on, and also some of those handicrafts take a bit of time and make a certain amount of mess.

Miss Laurio: Have you picked up any useful hints for teaching?

Miss Breckenridge: Something that came out of the Arnold-Forster history, when we asked the students to "tell the history of 'F.D.' on a penny." We got a lot of very good responses, telling all about Henry VIII as Defender of the Faith, and going into all kinds of other details about Henry's wives and Sir Thomas More and other things. It made me think of Kingsley's *Madam How and Lady Why*, where the father takes the boy out to look at a few scratches in a rock, and the whole thing turns into a story about glaciers moving across the earth. It seems that we overlook so many things…perhaps people too…that can really be so interesting if we take the time to find out more about them. Anyway, it seems like an excellent strategy for teaching to ask "Have you ever noticed that…" and give the story of why something is so, or to encourage the children to work it out for themselves if they can.

Miss White: What surprised you the most about this class?

Miss Breckenridge: The enthusiasm that they have for British geography! They seem to enjoy using Miss Mason's old *Geographical Readers*, even though some points have changed and do need to be corrected in class. Some of the students are quite expert already, and they do not falter much when it comes to names. Here's a response that was dictated by one of the nine-year-olds:

> Q. What towns, rivers, and castles would you see in travelling about Warwickshire?
>
> B. Warwick, Kenilworth, Coventry, Stratford, Leamington, and Birmingham are all towns which you would see if you travelled through Warwick.
> The Avon stretches from north to south of Warwickshire. It has its tributary the Learn, upon which Leamington is situated.
> There is a castle of Warwick and Coventry and Kenilworth. Warwick is the capital of the county. It has a famous castle, whose high and lofty towers stand upon the bank of the river Avon. Coventry is a very old town. It also has a beautiful castle, where the fair Lady Godiva and her father used to live.
> Stratford is called 'The Swan on the Avon,' because that is where Shakespeare, the great poet, was born and died, and this is a little

> piece of poetry about him; —
>
> 'Where his first infant lays, sweet Shakespeare sung,
> Where the last accents faltered on his tongue.'
>
> The river Avon takes its rise in the vale of Evesham, then winds through pleasant fields and meadows till it comes to the south of Warwickshire, and then it becomes broad and stately and flows on up to Coventry...

And so on.

Miss White: I see that boy as a future tour guide.

Study 23: The Middle Years

Miss Glass: Miss Capehart and Miss White, how are things going in the Form III class?

Miss White: I find the age grouping of eleven or twelve to fifteen interesting, as it does not exactly match anything we have right now in Canada; in our schools, those who finish Grade Eight would be about fourteen, and many do not go on to the High School classes. But I have heard that there will soon be something called Junior High Schools in the United States, and that sounds very much like Form III.

Miss Capehart: I'm sure you are all familiar with the subjects by this time, but here is the list:

Bible Lessons and Recitations (Poetry and Bible passages)
English Grammar, French, German, Italian, and Latin
English, French, and Ancient History (Plutarch's *Lives*)
Singing (French, English, and German Songs)
Writing, Dictation, Drill
Drawing in Brush and Charcoal
Natural History, Botany, Physiology, Geography
Arithmetic, Geometry
Reading

Miss White: The students in the correspondence school are allowed to make one or two subjects optional, such as Italian, especially for health reasons or if they have other outside lessons; but those coming to the Practicing School do *all* the work set, and their work compares satisfactorily with the rest, even though they have the disadvantage of changing teachers frequently. Though we see errors in many of their papers, they are not often the mistakes of ignorance, nor are they those of a person who has never understood what he is writing about.

Miss Capehart: Sometimes we have the mistaken notion that the greater the number of subjects the heavier the work; though, in reality, the contrary is the case, unless the hours of study are increased.

Miss White: The school day does seem quite a bit longer at this stage, as we are up to three and a half hours per day, with half an hour of that for drill and games. But the students do not have to prepare essay papers or do mathematics practice after they go home; they do their writing and so on during class time. And they are expected to write all their examinations by now, instead of dictating them.

Miss Bruce: Are they being taught composition lessons?

Miss White: Composition is not taught as a subject; Miss Mason says that well-taught children compose as well-bred children behave—by the light of nature.

Miss Glass: Can you show us some examples of their writing?

Miss White: Not so much their *spontaneous* efforts–for that you will have to wait for the little magazine that I believe some of them are working on–but their classroom responses are also well done, even poetic. Here is one from Plutarch's *Life of Aristides*, by a student who is thirteen years old.

> Q. Show fully how Aristides acquired the title of "The Just." Why was it a strange title for a man in those days?
>
> D.: —Aristides acquired the title of "The Just" by his justice, and because he never did anything unjust in order to become rich or powerful. While many of the judges and chief men in Athens took bribes, he alone always refused to do so, and he also never spent the public money on himself. When, after having defeated the Persians, at Platae, the Greek States decided to have a standing army, it was Aristides who was sent round to settle how much each town should contribute. And he did this so fairly and well, that all the Greek States blessed and praised his arrangement. *[I'm leaving a bit out here because it's long.]*
>
> In all that he did Aristides was inflexibly Just, and many stories were told of his justice. Though he loved his country well, he would never do anything wrong to gain for Athens some advantage, and in all he did his one aim was justice, and his only ambition to be called "The Just." He was so just and good, that he was called the "most just man in Greece."
>
> In the times in which Aristides lived, men used to care more to be called great, rich, or powerful than just. Themistocles, the great rival

of Aristides, used to do all he could to become the first man in Athens, and rich as well as powerful. He did not hesitate to take bribes, and all he did for the Athenians was done with a view to making himself the head of the people, and the first man in the State. He used often to do unjust as well as cruel things in order to get his own ends.

It was the same with most other men who lived at this time, they preferred being rich, powerful or great, to being distinguished by the title of "The Just."'

Miss Bruce: That seems a very…just…description.

Miss White: I liked this one, also from a thirteen-year-old:

Q. Give a diagram of the eye, and explain how we see everything. (Book studied, Dr Schofield's *Physiology for Schools*.)

H.: —The eye can be likened to a camera, and the brain to the man behind the camera. The image enters at the hole, passes through the lens, is reflected on the plate, but the camera does not see, it is the man behind the camera who sees. In the same way, the image passes in at the pupil and through the lens, both sides of which are curved, and can be tightened or slackened according to the distance of the image. Then the image passes along the nerve of sight to the two bulbs in the brain which see.

If you hold a rounded glass between a sheet of paper and the image at the right distance (for the glass cannot tighten or slacken like our lens), you will see the image reflected upside-down on the paper. This is the way the lens acts. There is a small yellow spot a little below the middle of the back of the eye; here the sight is more acute, and so, though we can see lots of things at one time, we can only look at one thing at a time. There is a blind spot where the nerve enters the eye (which shows that the nerve of sight itself is blind) so that some part of every image is lost, like a black dot punched in it. But we are so used to it that we cannot see it.

Miss Capehart: They were also asked to describe their favourite scene in Scott's *Waverley*. Myrtle is one of the youngest in the class, and not a great speller, but she retold the scene very well.

Already Waverly (*sic*) could hear the distant shouts of the men calling to each other coming nearer and nearer. Soon he could distinguish the antlers of the deer moving towards the opening like a forest of trees stiped (*sic*) of their leaves. The sportsmen prepared themselves to give them a warm reception, and all were ready as the deer entered the valley.

> They looked very ferocious, as they advanced towards where Edward and the cheifs (*sic*) were standing and seemed as if they were determined to fight; the roes and weaker ones in the centre, and the bulls standing as if on defence. As soon as they came within range, some of the cheifs (sic) fired, and two or three deer came down. Waverly also had the good fortune (and also the skill) to bring down a couple and gain the aplause (*sic*) of the other sportsmen. But the herd was now charging furiously up the valley towards them. The order was given to lie down, as it was impossible to stem the coming wave of deer; but as it was given in Gaelic it conveyed no meaning to Edward's mind, and he remained standing.
>
> The heard (*sic*) was now not fifty yards from him; and in another minute he would have been trampled to death; but Maclvor at his own risk, jumped up and literaly (*sic*) dragged him to the ground just as the deer reached them. Edward had a sensation as if he was out in a severe hail storm, but this did not last long.
>
> When they had passed, and Edward attempted to rise, he found that besides a number of bruises he had also severely sprained his ancle (*sic*), and was unable to walk, or even stand. A shelter was soon made for him out of a plaid in which he was laid; and then Maclvor called the Highland doctor or herbalist, to attend him. The doctor approached Edward with every sign of humiliation, but before attending to his ancle, he insisted upon walking slowly round him several times, in the direction in which the sun goes, muttering at the same time a spell over him as he went, and though Waverly was in great pain he bad to submit to his foolery. Waverly saw to his great astonishment that Maclvor believed or seemed to believe in the old man's cantations (*sic*) At last, when he bad finished his spells, which he seemed to think more necessary than the dressing, he drew from his pocket a little packet of herbs, some of which he applied to the sprained ancle (*sic*) and after it had been bound up, Edward felt much relieved. He rewarded the doctor with some money, the value of which seemed to exceed his wildest imaginations, for he heaped so many blessings upon the head of Waverly that MacIvor said, "A hundred thousand curses on you," whereupon he stopped.

Miss Laurio: What have I missed? Now I have to read *Waverley*.

Miss Capehart: What surprised me a little this week was the oral lesson given to the Form III students in "Reading"—that is, how to read well aloud! That is a skill that, I think, every teacher should have as well.

Miss Bruce: What took place during the lesson?

Miss Capehart: They "warmed up" with some breathing exercises, and reviewed the reason that these are important. The teacher then had the students practice consonant and vowel sounds, by giving them sentences in which difficulties in pronunciation occur. They found these exercises quite enjoyable:

> m, en, n. A stricken maiden musing on a mountain was given from heaven man in mortal form.
> final t. A just knight felt a weight on his heart, and yet a sweet quiet rest was present when he went to meet the light.
> p, b. A path of prickly brambles, bordered by pure pale poppies, breathed peace between the broken beams.
> d. Touched by the hand that appeared from the cloud under which nodded the dead leaves.

Now you might have expected that the next step would be to have the students practice reading a chosen passage, in this case some lines from Tennyson's "Sir Galahad." But no, the *teacher* read it aloud first, and then asked the students to describe the mental pictures they had "drawn" during the reading. She then showed them a reproduction of Watts' painting by the same name, and asked them in what points the poet's and the artist's ideas coincide. So they had already had put some real thought into the imagery of the poem, and its ideas, before they attempted to read it themselves.

Miss Breckenridge: Miss White, would you honour us with a reading?

Miss White: I'll try.

> A maiden knight to me is given
> Such hope, I know not fear;
> I yearn to breathe the airs of heaven
> That often meet me here.
> I muse on joy that will not cease,
> Pure spaces clothed in living beams,
> Pure lilies of eternal peace,
> Whose odours haunt my dreams;
> And, stricken by an angel's hand,
> This mortal armour that I wear,
> This weight and size, this heart and eyes
> Are touched, are turned to finest air.
> The clouds are broken in the sky,
> And through the mountain walls
> A rolling organ-harmony
> Swells up, and shakes and falls.
> Then move the trees, the copses nod,
> Wings flutter, voices hover clear:
> 'O just and faithful knight of God!
> Ride on! the prize is near.'
> So pass I hostel, hall and grange;
> By bridge and ford, by park and pale,

All-armed I ride, whate'er betide,
Until I find the Holy Grail.

[Silent appreciation.]

Study 24: The Teen Years

Miss Capehart: Miss Glass, you are teaching the upper forms right now, are you not?

Miss Glass: Yes, I have just begun. I think you all know Miss McKellar, from the second-year teaching class, whom I am working alongside. She is more familiar with the upper form work than I am.

Miss Breckenridge: Welcome, Miss McKellar. Have a biscuit?

Miss McKellar: Thank you. Well, you know that almost all the students in our upper form classes are girls, as the boys have gone off to their own schools. They are usually in Form IV for two or three years, from fourteen or fifteen to seventeen, after which they are ready to specialize and usually do well. The literature, used to illustrate the history lessons, includes the reading of a good many books, and the German and French books, when possible, also illustrate the history studied. All the books (about forty) are of a different calibre from those used in the lower classes; they are books for intelligent students.

Miss Glass: The programme for Form IV is especially interesting; it adds Geology and Astronomy to the sciences studied, more advanced Algebra to the Mathematics, and sets the history of Modern Europe instead of French history. *[See Appendix C: Two History Lessons]*

Miss White: Can you explain what they are doing in Astronomy?

Miss Glass: I was asked to present a half-hour oral lesson to the class, and I set these as my objectives:.

1. To interest the pupils in studying the heavens for themselves.
2. To show where the planets may be looked for and how they may be recognized.
3. To help the pupils to apply their theoretical knowledge of the planets to explain the movements they can observe with the naked eye.
4. To exercise the reasoning powers.

Miss White: And what happened during the lesson?

Miss Glass: I first asked the students to describe the changes to be seen in the sky at night, and, excluding the apparent motion caused by the earth's rotation, to find out whether they have noticed and contrasted the constellations of fixed stars and the planets (wanderers). I let them tell which of the planets are visible to the naked eye, and asked whether they had noticed when and where are to be seen, at the present date, Jupiter, Saturn, and Mars, which are in Capricornus, Sagittarius, and Leo, respectively.

Miss White: What do you mean by "in" them? I am ashamed to say how ignorant I am of astronomy, though I am doing my best to catch up.

Miss Glass: Well, you know that planets move relative to the stars as they orbit the sun? Because most constellations are easy to recognize, with a little practice, they are a good reference point for finding other objects in the sky. So, right now Saturn is in Sagittarius, and Mars is in Leo.

We discussed the ways by which planets can be distinguished from stars: for example, their steady light; their size, in the case of Venus and Jupiter; their colour, in the case of Mars; their position, relative to known constellations; and their motion, which would be noticeable after successive observations. To enlarge on that last point, I asked the students to name planets whose orbits are within that of the earth and those whose orbits are outside ours. By the help of a diagram of the solar system, I got them to infer, from the nearness to the sun of Venus and Mercury, that these planets are never visible at midnight, but only just before sunrise and after sunset.

I wanted the students to recognize the advantage of knowing the constellations by sight. I showed them Philip's "Planisphere" (a handy tool!), and I had them find the portion of the heavens visible at 6 p.m. today, and indicate, both in the heavens and with respect to our landscape, the positions of Jupiter and Saturn. I also showed them how Mars may be looked for in the south, too, at about 6 o'clock in the morning.

Miss Bruce: You obviously have an optimistic idea of students' ability to waken at 6 o'clock in the morning.

Miss Glass: Well, some of them said they would try. In any case, to illustrate the idea of the motion of the planets, I showed them a diagram of the path of Venus among the constellations in 1868 (there's one in Lockyer's *Elementary Lessons in Astronomy*), and I got the pupils to notice how large a distance she travelled in one month, in order to induce them to make personal observations. Of course there is the problem that sometimes the planets seem to move backwards, and at other times they remain stationary, although that's really because we are viewing them from our own planet which is also in motion. It's easier to understand if you actually move around the room and make observations, so that's what we did.

Miss Capehart: Most interesting! Miss McKellar, can you tell us more about the books used in the upper forms?

Miss McKellar: The literature, used to illustrate the history lessons, includes the reading of a good many books, and the German and French books when possible also illustrate the history studied. All the books (about forty) are of a different calibre from those used in the lower classes; they are books for intelligent students. As teachers, we notice that due growth has taken place in the minds of the girls, both as regards judgment and power of appreciation. This new maturity is easy to see by the level of work they submit, for instance in this response to Carlyle's essay on Robert Burns (which is not easy reading). I'll read just a part of it, as it is quite long.

> Carlyle looked upon Burns as one of the nicest of men and greatest of poets; rather a weak man, perhaps, but covering all his faults with his genius and kindness of heart, clever and persevering, and basely neglected and shunned by his contemporaries. It is quite extraordinary to read the world famous poems of this poet, and to remember that he was a ploughman, and surrounded only by the most uneducated peasants and fellow-labourers, though, of course, the life of a ploughman in the hills of Scotland is far more likely to encourage poetry and reflection than the life of many a London dentist or hair-dresser far higher in rank; but it is easy to believe in fact, that Burns would have found inspirations for his genius in a flat sandy waste or a grocer's shop, and, as Carlyle says, a man or woman is not a genius unless they are extraordinary, not really inspired if such a person could have been imagined before. Robert Burns has provided Scotland for centuries at least, with plenty of national poetry, his poems are such as can be enjoyed, like flowers and trees and all things really beautiful, by old and young, stupid and clever, fishermen and prime ministers––surely that is a work of which any man would be proud!

Miss Glass: The students, by this time, are studying not only the grammar of English, but going deeper into its *nuances*. Here, just for fun, why don't we try their examination question from Trench's *Study of Words*?

> Q. Distinguish between arrogant and presumptuous, interference and interposition, genuine and authentic, hate and detest, loathe and abhor, education and instruction, apprehend and comprehend, using each word in a sentence. [*For the student response, see Appendix D.*]

Miss Capehart: The arrogant student corrected her teacher for misspelling something on the blackboard. The student's mother was presumptuous enough to come to the school and complain to the headmistress about the poor level of teaching her daughter was receiving.

Miss Breckenridge: Oh dear, did that really happen?

Miss Capehart: I am not naming names.

Miss Breckenridge: Interference and interposition? That's a bit difficult; can I use a past tense? Jack interposed himself between his two quarreling friends, but they told him not to interfere.

Miss White: Interposition can also mean something like intervention or mediation, is that not so? In that case I should think it would be a little less intrusive than interference.

Miss Breckenridge: But close in meaning, so that's not an easy one.

Miss Bruce: Genuine and authentic? Again, those seem very close in meaning. I would use genuine to refer to objects, but I suppose people could also be genuine, meaning honest, without guile. Authentic? That seems to imply that someone verified something to be genuine. I think I'm getting confused.

Miss McKellar: That one is difficult to get right unless you have studied the *Words* book. "Authentic" refers to something undisputed, such as the authentic letters of an author. "Genuine" has the more general meaning of true, real.

Miss White: Hate and detest, loathe and abhor? I'm sure I can't get all of those right. I loathe and detest porridge with lumps in it. I abhor racy novels. I hate to see a home without books. How did I do?

Miss Glass: Actually all four words can apply to people, which makes it more difficult. For instance, someone can be loathsome or detestable, but you don't truly hate the person, he is not your enemy.

Miss Laurio: And these students don't get arrogant because they think they know more about words than anyone else? Astounding. I'll try "education" and "instruction." You can receive instruction in knitting or gymnastics, but that doesn't give you an education. Everyone knows that education is…

Everyone: The science of relations.

Miss Glass: Miss McKellar, I'm looking at the student's response to this, and I think she got it backwards. This is what Trench says in the book:

> Thus, for instance, it often is with 'instruction' and 'education,' Cannot we 'instruct' a child, it is asked, cannot we teach it geography, or arithmetic, or grammar, quite independently of the Catechism, or even of the Scriptures? No doubt you may; but can you 'educate' without bringing moral and spiritual forces to bear upon the mind and affections of the child? And you must not be

> permitted to transfer the admissions which we freely make in regard of 'instruction,' as though they also held good in respect of 'education.' For what is 'education'? Is it a furnishing of a man from without with knowledge and facts and information? or is it a drawing forth from within and a training of the spirit, of the true humanity which is latent in him? Is the process of education the filling of the child's mind, as a cistern is filled with waters brought in buckets from some other source? or the opening up for that child of fountains which are already there? Now if we give any heed to the word 'education,' and to the voice which speaks therein, we shall not long be in doubt. Education must educe, being from 'educare,' which is but another form of 'educere'; and that is to draw out, and not to put in. 'To draw out' what is in the child, the immortal spirit which is there, this is the end of education; and so much the word declares. The putting in is indeed most needful, that is, the child must be instructed as well as educated, and 'instruction' means furnishing; but not instructed instead of educated. He must first have powers awakened in him, measures of value given him; and then he will know how to deal with the facts of this outward world; then instruction in these will profit him; but not without the higher training, still less as a substitute for it.

Miss McKellar: I believe you're right; I'll have to make a note of that.

Miss Breckenridge: Still, that's a lot to comprehend.

Study 25: What is an Oral Lesson?

Miss Laurio: Miss McKellar, while you are here, might I ask for some clarification on the matter of "oral lessons?" I understood, from our study of Herbart and so on, that teachers were not required to "get up" a lesson; and I have heard Miss Mason say that the teacher must not get between the child and the book. What then is the purpose of these oral lessons that we are required to plan?

Miss McKellar: You're correct, that the part of the teacher, even of younger children, should be something like a University tutor who "reads with" his students. However, we do schedule special lessons for various purposes: sometimes to introduce a course of reading, or in bringing certain readings to a point. These lessons are always expansions or illustrations or summaries of some part of the scholars' current book-work. They also give an opportunity for the teacher to read passages from various books bearing on the subject on hand

Miss White: How does that differ from a lecture?

Miss McKellar: The lecture, as we usually think of it, is accompanied by note-taking, and is expected to be followed up by reports. The oral lesson can be thought of as a channel for free intellectual sympathy between "teacher and taught," and a means of widening the intellectual horizon of children. And some subjects, such as Languages, Mathematics, and Science, depend largely upon oral teaching and demonstrations, so it is important that we plan such lessons as will open that channel.

Here are the notes for an oral lesson I gave to the students of the upper forms, which introduced Charles Lamb's *Essays of Elia*, but which also touched on some principles to guide the choice of reading, and to emphasize the fact that very thoughtful reading is necessary in order to get full pleasure and benefit from a book. I should explain that the students were already familiar with some of the essays, and knew a bit about the life of Charles Lamb, so I wanted to draw on that knowledge.

> Step 1. Decide *with the pupils* as to some principles which should guide us in the choice of books, such as the following:
>
> Never waste time on valueless books.
> *Have respect for the books themselves.*
> Try to cultivate taste by noticing the best passages in any book that is being read.
> *Time is too short to read much; there is a necessity, therefore, for judicious selection.*
> The best literature can only be appreciated by those who have fitted themselves for it.
> *It is more important to read well than to read much.*
> The gain of reading some of the most beautiful literature while we are young is that we shall then have beautiful thoughts and images to carry with us through life.
> *To get at the full significance of a book it is necessary to dig for it.*
>
> Thus the *Essays of Elia* are not only pleasant reading, but they are the reflection of the writer's character. All that Charles Lamb was can be gathered from his works, and to rightly understand these one must know something of his grand though obscure life.
>
> Step 2. Brief outline of Charles Lamb's life (given as much as possible by the students themselves).
>
> I read them some thoughts by Lamb's editor Thomas Noon Talfourd. I also noted that Lamb's letters to Robert Lloyd show Lamb's persistent cheerfulness. This cheerful tone is also noticeable in many of his essays, of which I pointed out a few examples.
>
> Step 3. Summarize the lesson by questions.

Miss Laurio: Can you give us an example of how that is done with a younger class?

Miss McKellar: Yes, here are my notes for an Old Testament lesson.

Group: History. Class lb. Average age: 8.
Time: 20 minutes.

OBJECTS.

1. To so interest the children in the story of Jacob's death, that they may not forget it.
2. To give a new idea of God as drawn from the story of Jacob's deathbed :—God's abiding presence.
3. To give them an admiration for Joseph as one who honoured his father and mother.

LESSON.

Step I. Recapitulate the former lesson, and follow Jacob's journeying with his family from Canaan to Egypt, on a map.

Step 2. Show the children how Joseph was the first of Jacob's sons to visit him when he was ill. Draw their attention to the particular trait of Joseph's character shown in this story.

Step 3. Describe in a few words the surroundings in which the events of the story take place.

Step 4. Read carefully to the children suitable parts of Genesis xlviii., reminding them to pay special attention to the words of the Bible, as they so beautifully express the scene.

Step 5. While the children are narrating in the words of the Bible, help them by questions to bring out the important points of the story.

Step 6. Help the children to realize how Joseph's love of his father affected his life, and how they should let their parents feel their love.

Step 7. Let the children see that this family realized God's abiding presence, and show them how any family can realize it in the same way, if it will.

Miss Breckenridge: How are these principles applied in, say, a handicraft class, or some other lesson on *things* rather than *books*?
[Bell rings]

Miss McKellar: Oh, I need to run to class myself. But here are some of my other notes; I hope they will answer your questions.

Oral Lesson Notes

Subject: Design.

Division: Art. Class IV. Average age: 16 1/2.
Time: 40 minutes.

OBJECTS.

1. To give the girls an idea of how to fill a space decoratively, basing the design on a given plant.
2. To show them that good ornament is taken from nature, but a mere copy of nature to decorate an object is not necessarily ornamental.
3. To give them an appreciation of good ornament and help them to see what is bad.
4. To draw out their originality by letting them make designs for themselves.
5. If possible, to give them a taste for designing by giving them some ideas as to its use.

LESSON.

Step 1. Ask the girls what is meant by a design.

Step 2. After getting from them as much as possible, explain to them that a design is not a mere copy from nature, although it should be true to nature; make them see this by simply copying a plant in a required space to be designed (let this space be for a book cover). It will look meaningless and uninteresting, and does not fill the space, therefore it will not be ornamental. Then show the girls that a design requires thought and invention in arranging it to ornament the object.

Step 3. Point out to them that the most beautiful designs and those that have had the most thought spent upon them are the most simple. Show examples of this in Greek Ornament—Greek Honeysuckle, Egg and Dart Moulding.

Step 4. Tell the pupils that you wish them to make a design for a linen book cover, 7 by 5 inches, and if they have not time to finish to go on with it at home; if they like to carry the design out practically, to transfer it to linen and work it.

Step 5. Show the girls the flower from which they are to take their design, and point out its characteristics—the general growth of the plant, the curves which it makes, the form of the flower and leaves, and the way the leaves are joined to the central stem; these characteristics should not be lost sight of, but be made use of in giving character to the design, and treated as simply as possible.

Step 6. Let them begin their designs first of all by construction lines, and then clothe them with flowers and leaves, seeing that the masses are in good proportion. If time permits the design could be tinted in two colours, one for the background representing the linen, and the other for the pattern upon it.

Step 7. Suggest to them different ways in which they can make use of design in making simple patterns for their handicrafts, such as leather-work, wood-carving, and brass-work.

Subject: Cooking.

Division: Handicrafts. Class IV.
Time. 45 minutes.

OBJECTS.

1. To teach the students to make little cakes.
2. To show them that cooking must have method in it.
3. To give them opportunity of thinking for themselves why certain things should be done.
4. To show them how they can alter a recipe to make it richer or plainer.
5. To interest them in cooking.

LESSON

Step 1. Show the students how to manage the stove for cooking.
Step 2. Show them all the utensils to be used, and let them arrange them on the table.
Step 3. Let them write out the recipe from dictation.
Step 4. Let them grease the tins first with melted butter. Then let them each weigh out the ingredients on pieces of kitchen paper, and let them work independently of each other, the teacher also doing the same thing, so that the pupils may be able to see how to set to work without having their own work interfered with. During the process ask them why certain things should be done—for instance, why baking powder should be used, why the patty-pans should be greased. Tell them that if they wished to make the cakes plainer they could use milk instead of eggs, or if richer, they could add raisins and currants and spice. When the mixture is beaten and put into the patty-pans, let the students put them into the oven.
Step 5. After cleaning up the kitchen together, let the students see for themselves if the cakes are done; they should be a light brown. Then let them place them on a sieve to cool, and then arrange them on plates for the table.

Notes for a New Era

With Folded Hands...Or Not

As a young mother, my church-going kit for three young children included picture books, soft toys, and oatie-O's, which drew verbal criticism from an older gentleman sitting behind us. Church-behaviour norms, as he felt free to point out, had slipped badly since his childhood (probably spent in the same pew).

In a post on *The Hedgehog Review* blog, Alan Jacobs (2022b) writes that "Human beings are extremely skilled at recognizing and internalizing the norms of any given medium or environment," and that these norms "can alter over time." What does this mean? Think of what you might have read about the original audiences for Shakespeare's plays: they tended to be much rowdier than today's theater patrons. Another example Jacobs mentions, echoing my own experience, is how people are expected to conduct themselves during church services—and that can vary a great deal, even in the Middle Ages, when it was not uncommon for people to play cards during Mass. In some cultures, it's common for people to arrive late for worship services, and to go in and out as they like; of course, in those same cultures, sermons can go on for quite a while. In some churches, it's acceptable to clap, or shout, or dance; but not in others. The point of all this, as Jacobs points out, is that "at any given moment in time most people know what the attentional [and behavioural] norms are for any social endeavor they participate in." More or less, of course.

Jacobs' real concern is that, due to events of the past few years which have required many of us to make use of videoconferencing for one thing or another (and another and another), our standards of group or audience behaviour have shifted; and that makes it harder for speakers or teachers to know if their message is being heard. Listeners tune in and out not only mentally, but literally; they turn off audio or video to deal with interruptions, or type on another device while in the meeting, without feeling we have to explain or apologize (unless it's a very small group). As a lecturer, Jacobs finds this apparent lack of attention difficult to handle, so he prefers to record himself speaking, have students comment about it through a forum or email, and then record another video responding to those questions and comments.

But this is what I found most interesting about Jacobs' complaints:

> My instructions lack the force that habituation enjoys. The only way that I could address this problem would be to pause—and to pause often—in the midst of whatever I am saying to tell someone to come back and pay attention. But, of course, in many cases the person wouldn't be able to hear me, and my interjections would be so frequent that there would be less and less of substance in the class session to be inattentive *to*. Again: Such interjections would *have* to be frequent because I lack the power to reset the attentional norms that have recently, but firmly, taken hold...And while the norms of

> any particular moment are in a sense not objectively good or bad, they can be good or bad in relation to certain human purposes. The purposes I have in my classes are not compatible with the attentional norms that we've learned to employ in our teleconferencing pandemic. (Jacobs, 2022b)

Did you catch a couple of details there? "I lack the power to reset the attention norms that have...taken hold." As a university lecturer, or preacher, or teacher of adults, one also has certain norms of behaviour, and scolding the group for lack of attention, as one might a circle of preschoolers, is not acceptable. One is also not expected to use cute devices such as "I'm not going to begin until I see *everyone's* eyes looking at me." In a culture with such rapidly changing etiquette, it is (as Jacob says) largely on the speaker or teacher to work within those new norms; to find creative and respectful ways of encouraging attentiveness, while admitting that not everyone will be tuned in all of the time.

However, in a Charlotte Mason-inspired school classroom, it may be understood that we meet for a purpose, and that those purposes are simply not compatible with inattention. We come together for the real work of learning, and that is taken as seriously for a young child as it is for one about to graduate. Does it mean that students looking out the window should be scolded? That we should close the curtains? Does that mean that children (particularly in a homeschool setting) must sit with folded hands during a reading, rather than doodle or play with blocks or even jump up and down on a trampoline? No, but it might mean that we try to minimize noise and other non-useful distractions.

Does it mean that teachers (or preachers, or other speakers) need to become entertainers? No, we do not need to set messages to music or speak them through puppets or animated videos, if the words are worthwhile in themselves. And if they're not, no amount of showmanship is going to make them so. However...the further our audience is from the "habituation" of attention, because they are still *learning* the habit, or because they never *had* it, or even because it has been more recently *lost* in these normative shifts, the more creative we may have to be with breaking up long readings; in giving listeners extra opportunities to respond (or narrate); or in confirming, without being patronizing, that the important points have been heard. We need to spread the feast; but learning still needs to take place in the mind of the student.

And that is why Charlotte Mason's emphasis on *books* and *things*, and her de-emphasis on Herbartian "getting up a lesson," takes some of that pressure and anxiety off the teacher—even in the twenty-first century; and even if we must speak on a virtual platform. We do not rule by punishment, but we do recognize authority; and we do not demand folded hands, but we do value attention.

(Did you get all that down?)

Part Six: My Dear Margaret (or, Consider All the Aspects)

Idleness was a cardinal sin in the Stirling household. When Valancy had been a child she had been made to write down every night, in a small, hated, black notebook, all the minutes she had spent in idleness that day. On Sundays her mother made her tot them up and pray over them. (L.M. Montgomery, *The Blue Castle*)

First let us consider the principle of authority, which is the basis of moral as it is of religious teaching. 'Ought' is part of the verb 'to owe,' and that which we owe is a personal debt to a Lawgiver and Ruler, however men name the final authority. If they choose to speak of Buddha or Humanity, they do not escape from the sense of a moral authority. They know that that which they *ought* is that which they owe to do, a debt to some power or personality external to themselves... To us, who know the name of God and have the revelation of the Scriptures, authority carries no vague terror. We know what is required of us, and that the requirements are never arbitrary, but necessary in the nature of things, both for the moral government of the world and to gratify the unquenchable desire of every human soul to rise into a higher state of being. Perhaps parents, great as they are and should be in the eyes of their children, should always keep well to the front the fact that their authority is derived. (*School Education*, p. 126)

Study 26: Aspects of Physical Training

In these letters, Miss Mason addresses herself to her niece Margaret, offering her opinion on many aspects of child-raising, but attempting not to vex her too much with unasked-for advice.

June 16, 1904

My dear Margaret,

How lovely it was to see you all in London this past week, and what a good time the children seem to have had in viewing the Trooping the Colour! Philip in particular seemed quite taken with the soldiers. It would be good work to keep to the front this idea of living under authority, training under authority, serving under authority, a discipline of life readily self-embraced by children, in whom the heroic impulse is always strong. It is well that a child should be taught to "keep under his body and bring it into subjection" (1 Cor. 9:27), first, to the authority of his parents and, later, to the authority of his own will (you knew I would come to that eventually!); and always, because no less than this is due, to the divine Authority in whom he has his being.

In your last letter to me you described your new plan of health and physical training, and the splendid exercise equipment which you have planned to purchase for the children. While I applaud your desire to provide them with healthy bodies, may I gently suggest that you consider some of its deeper aspects? Perhaps never since the days of the Olympian games has more attention been paid to physical culture than it receives in England to-day. But possibly this physical cult suffers from the want of unity and sanctity of purpose which nullifies to a considerable extent most of our educational efforts. In other words, dear Margaret, does our culture's new *mania* for physical perfection create real heroes? and this was the object of physical culture among the early Greeks, anyway. Men must be heroes, or how could they fulfil the heavy tasks laid upon them by the gods? Heroes are not made in a day; therefore, the boy was trained from his infancy in heroic exercises, and the girl brought up to be the mother of heroes.

We want to turn out "a fine animal," a man or woman with a fine physique and in good condition, and we get what we lay ourselves out for. If we visit historic homes and museums, we are often surprised at the shortness of the beds, or the seeming smallness of the preserved garments: so it seems true that we are bigger, stronger, and perhaps healthier, or at least longer-lived, than our forebears. So far, so good, and young Philip and Beatrice will undoubtedly surpass their Great-Aunt Charlotte in height before long.

But the object of the fine physical culture that English youths and maidens receive is, too often, the poor and narrow one that they may get the most, especially the most of physical enjoyment, out of life; and so young people "train their bodies to hardships" (1 Cor. 9:27), and pamper them with ease and self-indulgence by turns, the one and the other being for their own pleasure: the pampering being the more delightful after the period of training, and the training itself rather a pleasant change from the softness of pampering. Now it is true that some young people prefer to endure hardness all the time, and go off in the Berserker spirit (do you remember your Viking stories?) to find adventures; but even this is not the best that might be done.

The object of athletics and gymnastics should be kept steadily to the front; enjoyment is good by the way, but is not the end; the end is the preparation of a body, available from crown to toe, for whatever behest "the gods" may lay upon us. "Ye *are* your own," is perhaps the unspoken thought of most young persons—if they are their own, they must be free to do as they like *with* their own. But excess in sports, excess in easy-going pleasure, excess in study, excess in random reading, excess of carelessness in regard to health, any excess that we have a mind to, is lawful to us if only it serves as the means to an end. This loose morality with regard to our physical debts, without touching actual *vice*, which is probably on the decline, is the reason why the world does not get all that it should out of such splendid material.

And lest you accuse this old woman of being a wet blanket, I would not reduce the pleasures of childhood and youth by an iota; rather I think this would *increase* them, for the disciplined life has more power of fresh enjoyment than is given to the unrestrained. And of course we no longer think that it is character-building or wholesome to deny our children their real physical needs. All we claim is that every young person shall be brought up under the sense of authority in the government, management, and training of his body. The sense that health is a duty, and that any trifling with health, whether vicious or careless, is really of the nature of *suicide*, springs from this view—that life is held in trust from a supreme Authority.

But to bring ourselves under authority at all times would require a constantly repeated effort of thought and which would make life too laborious. Authority must be sustained by habit! Can you stand to read a few reminders about that old "hobby" of mine? I promise to limit my thoughts on it to on our subject of physical training. Well, you know what I have said before about habits: that frequently-repeated thoughts or acts leave some sort of register or mark in the brain tissue which tends to make the repetition of such thoughts at first easy, and at last automatic. In all matters of physical exercise it is obvious to us that—do a thing a hundred times and it becomes easy; do a thing a thousand times and it becomes mechanical, as easy to do as not. This principle is abundantly applied in cricket, boating, golf, cycling, all the "labours" we delight in.

But there is an outfit of half-physical, half-moral habits of life which the playing-field tends to form, but which are apt to be put on and off with the sporting clothes if they are not steadily and regularly practised in the home life also. These are the habitudes which it is the part of parents to give their children, and, indeed, they do form part of the training of all well brought-up young people, so I am sure that you have not been neglecting this either; but it is well not to lose sight of this part of our work. For instance, self-restraint in seemingly harmless pleasures, such as over-indulging in sweets or snacks, or allowing too frequent lethargic, self-indulgent intervals, such as "lounging" in an arm-chair with a novel. Remember that we are talking here about the discipline of physical training, with a real end in view, and about the building of young heroes—so the majority of their amusements should be healthful, and their occupations should be profitable. The American writer Lydia Maria Child once wrote,

> Provided brothers and sisters go together, and are not allowed to go with bad children, it is a great deal better for the boys and girls on a farm to be picking blackberries at six cents a quart, than to be wearing out their clothes in useless play. They enjoy themselves just as well, and they are earning something to buy clothes, at the same time they are tearing them.

Yes, I thought you would enjoy that one. Well, I will stop there for now, and I send you all my love.

Yours affectionately…

June 22, 1904

My dear Margaret,

No, I am not at all saying that every moment of a child or young person's time must be accounted for. Boys and girls must have time to invent episodes, carry on adventures, live heroic lives, lay sieges and carry forts, even if the fortress be an old armchair; and in these affairs the elders must neither meddle nor make. Adults must be content to know that they do not understand, and, what is more, that they carry with them a chill breath of reality which sweeps away illusions. Think what it must mean to a general in command of his forces to be told by some intruder into the play-world to tie his shoe-strings!

I am also not particularly recommending that they take up ugly or unnecessary handicrafts just to keep their hands from being idle. But as little as you may think of that crewelwork picture your grandmother made, the work was probably better for her morally and physically than the relaxed muscles and mind of an equal time spent lounging with a library book.

So we have said something about self-restraint in too-frequent indulgences, as something that we expect children to cultivate for themselves. What about the other "self" habits, self-control and self-discipline? You will say that they all sound much the same, and perhaps you will come up with better names, but here is what I mean:

Self-control: This can take many forms, but we most often recognize someone with good self-control as the one who is most level-headed in emergencies, and also one who can maintain a cheerful attitude, who does not fuss about small inconveniences, who does not push to be first in line—indeed, this is a habit which should be trained in the nursery. "If you are vexed, don't show it," is usually quite safe teaching, because every kind of fretfulness, impatience, resentfulness, nervous irritability generally, grows with expression and passes away under self-control. It is worthwhile to remember that the physical signs promote mental state just as much as the mental state causes the physical signs.

Self-discipline: The discipline *of* habit is never complete until it becomes self-discipline *in* habits. It is not a trifle that even the nursery child spills his milk, breaks his playthings, dawdles about his small efforts. The well-trained child delights to bring himself into good habits in these respects. Philip knows that to be cleanly, neat, prompt, orderly, is so much towards making a man of him, and "man" and "hero" are in his thought synonymous terms. Habits of behaviour; habits of deportment, habits of address, tones of voice, etc., all the habits of a gentleman-like bearing and a kind and courteous manner, fall under this head of self-discipline in bodily habits. (And of course we can use less masculine terms if Beatrice insists…perhaps you will come up with some unique word that your children understand to mean the same thing.)

Of course I am not suggesting that you turn your children into little prigs *[Study 15]*, but you should also feel satisfied that their training will stand them in good stead even when they are away from home.

And as I'm sure that you've had enough meddling and lecturing, no matter how well meant, I will end off for now. Give my love to the young fry,

Yours affectionately…

June 30, 1904

My dear Margaret,

In my last letter I listed some habitudes of *body*, which become, also, *mental* and *moral* habitudes:

Self-control in emergencies,
Self-restraint in indulgences, and
Self-discipline in habits.

You asked (I hope seriously) if there are any others. Yes, I can think of one or two more: alertness to seize opportunities; promptness and vigour in bodily exercises; and quick perception as to that which is to be seen, heard, felt, tasted, smelt.

As for encouraging children in seizing possibly rare opportunities, particularly for doing some little service, or some piece of courtesy—this is something that you will never regret as a parent. It is well to bring up children to think it is rather a sad failure if they miss a chance of delivering a message, opening a door, carrying a parcel, any small act of service that presents itself.

They should be taught to be equally alert to seize opportunities of getting knowledge; it is the nature of children to regard each grown-up person they meet as a fount of knowledge on some particular subject; so let their training keep up the habit of eager inquiry. Success in life depends largely upon the cultivation of alertness to seize opportunities, and this is largely a *physical* habit.

Closely connected with that alertness is the habit of quick perception as to all that is to be seen, heard, felt, tasted, smelt in a world gives illimitable information through our five gateways of knowledge. I am sure that you can devise games and tasks that will give opportunity to develop those, as also with the habits I mentioned of physical exercise. Do remember, though, that as children learn to discriminate with their senses, they should be discouraged from using merely judgmental words such as "horrid," but should be limited to descriptive words such as "bitter," and comparative terms such as "taller than Papa." The only other point I can urge is that the quickness of observation natural to the children should not be taken for granted; in time, and especially as school studies press upon them, they may seem to lose their early quickness at such things; but the trained habit of seeing all that is to be seen, hearing all that is to be heard, remains through life.

But, while we think of the physical habits that become mental ones, what of the reverse? A habit becomes morally binding in proportion to the inspiring power of the *idea* which underlies it. You ask for an example? *Fortitude* is one. Touch the right spring and children are capable of an amazing amount of steady effort. I know a little boy of ten who set himself the task of a solitary race of three miles every day in the hot summer holidays because he was to compete in a race when he went back to school; and this, not because he cared much about sports, but because his eldest brother had always distinguished himself in them, and he must do the same.

When we think how little power we have to do the tiresome things we set ourselves to do every day, we appreciate the compelling power a child can use, given a strong enough impulse. The long name, Fortitude, would have its effect on your young Philip and Beatrice in the dentist's hands. It is good to know that it is a "manly" and "knightly" virtue to be strong to bear pain and inconvenience without making any sign. (Along with the other virtues such as service, courage, prudence, and chastity.)

But praying, as their fond great-aunt, that all the necessary repairs will be made without excessive pain to them! Much love to all,

Yours affectionately…

Study 27: Aspects of Intellectual Training

July 10, 1904

My dear Margaret,

We all recognize that we are under the reign of law so far as our bodies go. We know that "put your finger in the fire and it will be burnt," "sit in a draught and you will catch cold" (how is dear little Beatrice, by the way? I hope she will soon be back to her sunny self); "live a vigorous and temperate life and health will be your reward." That law attends our steps, with its penalties and rewards in all matters physical, we know very well.

Some of us go further and have a personal sense of the Lawgiver in matters of sickness and health. In sickness especially we feel that God is dealing with us, and we endeavour to lay ourselves open to the lesson of the hour. In moral matters, too, we live "under the law." We may forget ourselves, but we have compunctions, scruples; we are aware of penalties.

But in matters *intellectual* we are disposed to stand upon our rights. Every man is free to his own opinion, however casually formed. Every man kindles his own "lights," and thinks that no more is expected of him than to live up to those lights. In fact our attitude with regard to our own intellectual processes leads to that disturbing sense of *duality* which causes the shipwreck of many lives, the distressing unrest of others, and the easy drifting of many more.

Our thinking is not a separate thing from our conduct and our prayers, or even from our bodily well-being. A human being is not several entities. He or she is one spirit (visibly expressed in bodily form), with many powers. He or she can work and love and pray and live righteously, but all these are the outcome of the manner of thoughts (s)he thinks. And that, dear Margaret, is (like the other matters), the law, the authority, under which we live and teach and raise our children.

And, as in the other matters, we commit offenses against the law, and oppose ourselves to authority—in two directions, particularly. In the first place we are disposed to regard everything by turns as an open question. We forget that there are three ultimate postulates which the thought of man can neither prove nor disprove, though in every age it has played uneasily about one or the other. God, Self, and the World, are the three fixed points of thought. The active Western mind, with each new evolution of scientific thought, finds again and again that there is no place for God in the world; nay, so active and pleasant is the conception of *self* that an important school of philosophy has demonstrated that the real world is no more than a simulacrum, a *mirage*, as it were, projected from the conscious *self*. (The Eastern mind, is, on the contrary, inclined to regard selfhood as a passing phase in a state of absorption or reabsorption by deity.) But when we learn to realize that–God *is*, Self *is*, the World *is*, with all that these existences imply, quite untouched by any thinking of ours, unprovable, and self-proven,–we are at once put into a more humble attitude of mind. We recognize that above us, about us, within us, there are (as Hamlet says) "more things . . . than are dreamt of in our philosophy." We realize ourselves as persons; we have a local habitation; and we live and move and have our being in and under a supreme authority. It is not well we should take it for granted that everybody knows these things. Perhaps we all have a hearsay acquaintance with, but very few of us have a realizing knowledge of, these ultimate facts.

A second direction in which it is well that we should recognize our limitations is with regard to the nature and function of what we call our reason, and should, perhaps, describe more accurately as our power of reasoning. We all know how often we go to bed with a difficult question to settle. We say we will sleep upon it, and, in the morning, behold, the whole question has worked itself into shape: we see all its bearings and know just how to act. We are so accustomed to take wonders as matters of course, mere everyday events, that it does not occur to us to be surprised. We even say, the mind is clearer after sleep, regardless of the fact that we have no labour of thinking at all in the morning; all comes straight of itself. When we come to think of it, most of our decisions arrive in this unlaborious way. We really cannot say that we have thought such and such a matter out: the decision comes to us "in a flash," "by an intuition," what you will.

The subject is a large one, but all I care to stipulate for here is that children should be taught to know that much of our reasoning and so-called thinking is involuntary,–
–is as much a natural function as is the circulation of our blood, and that *this very fact* points to the *limitations* of Reason.

You did not expect that that was what I would say next?

All the same, it is something to think about...if you will pardon the expression.

Yours affectionately...

July 19, 1904

My dear Margaret,

No, what I said in my last letter (about the limitations of Reason) does not mean that we should not use Reason, or that what I have always told you about the Way of Reason is false. But all that Reason does for us is to prove, logically, any idea we choose to entertain.

For example, as I have said, important schools of philosophy (both Eastern and Western) entertain the idea that there is no actual real world independent of man's conception thereof. The logical proofs of this premise pour in upon their minds in such volume that a considerable literature exists to *prove an idea* which on the face of it appears absurd. We all know that if we entertain a notion that a servant is dishonest, that a friend is false, that a dress is unbecoming, well then some power within us, unconsciously to us, sets to work to collect evidence and bring irrefragable, indisputable *proof* of the position we have chosen to take up. This is the story of *Othello*, and of King Solomon's turning against David. It is the history of wars and persecutions and family feuds all over the world.

How necessary then that a child should be instructed to understand the limitations of his own reason! so that he will not confound logical demonstration with eternal truth, and will know that the important thing to him is the ideas he permits himself to entertain, and not by any means the *conclusions* he draws from these ideas, because these latter are self-evolved.

I had forgotten to mention a third fallacy which lies at the root of our thinking, and therefore, of our education, is, that while nature, morals, and theology may be more or less divine in their origin and relations, not only is *intellect* man's proper and peculiar sphere, but *knowledge*,—the knowledge of witty inventions, of man and nature, of art and literature, of the heavens above and the earth beneath,—all this knowledge is man's proper discovery. (Oh my dear Margaret—no jokes please about the male vs. the female intellect. You know your aunt cannot always be teased to take the time to write "him or her," and "Man" is still a serviceable word for "Person.")

Now did you read that carefully, over your laughter? *Intellect* and *knowledge* are our particular birthright. We have found it out ourselves, thought it out for ourselves, observed, reasoned, collected, laboured, gathered our forces, altogether of our own will and for our own ends and as independent agents.

Now, this pride of intellect also comes of the arrogance of man; not only in our age (which, I venture to think, is the very best age the world has ever seen), but in all time. It is our nature to lift up our heads and say, "We are the people; before us there were none like unto us, neither shall there be any more after us" (Joel 2:2).

But when we "come to ourselves," as the Prodigal Son did, we realize that our Author (think of that! Authority!) and Father has not in this way made over any single vast realm of our lives into our own hands. The knowledge that comes to us is given us in feasts, so to speak (as per the Prodigal Son). Great eras of scientific discovery or literary activity or poetic insight or artistic interpretation come to the world from time to time; and then there is a long interval for the assimilation of the new knowledge or the new thought. After that, the world is taken by storm by the rise of another constellation of its great intellects; and yet we do not discern the signs of the times (Matt. 16:3), nor realize that thus our God is bringing *us* up in knowledge, which is also divine, just as much as in the "nurture and admonition of the Lord" (Ephesians 6:4).

The medieval Church recognized this great truth—as Mr. Ruskin has eloquently pointed out, showing how the "Captain Figures," the inventors, as it were, of grammar and music, astronomy and geometry, arithmetic and logic, all spake that which was in them under the direct outpouring of the Holy Spirit, even though none of them had any such revelation of the true God as we recognize *[Study 10]*. What a revolution should we have in our methods of education if we could once conceive that dry-as-dust subjects like grammar and arithmetic should come to children, living with the life of the Holy Spirit, who, we are told, "shall teach you all things."

Yours affectionately…

P.S. It may occur to you to consider that such lines of thought as I have suggested are perhaps interesting but not practical. Believe me, nothing is so practical as a great idea, because nothing produces such an abundant outcome of practical effort. We must not turn the cold shoulder to philosophy. And education is no more than applied philosophy—our effort to train children according to the wisdom that is in us; and not according to the last novelty in educational ideas.

July 27, 1904

My dear Margaret,

And what about the formation of intellectual habits?

That need not occupy us long. We know that the possession of some half-dozen such habits makes up what is well called *ability*. They make a person able to do that which he desires to do with his mental powers, and to labour at the cost of not a tenth part of the waste of tissue which the same work would exact of a person of undisciplined mental habits. We know, too, that the habits in question are acquired through training and are not bestowed as a gift. Genius itself, we have been told, is an infinite capacity for taking pains; we would rather say, is the habit of taking infinite pains, for every child is born with the capacity.

But how do we get ourselves—or our children—able to make full use of those mental habits? Teachers trust–perhaps a little blindly–to the training which certain subjects give in certain mental habits. The classics, we consider, cultivate in one direction, the mathematics, in another, science, in a third. So they do, undoubtedly, so far as each of these subjects is concerned; but possibly not in forming the *general* habits of intellectual life which we expect to result. Remove the mathematician from his own field and he is not more exact or more on the spot than other men; indeed he is rather given to make a big hole for the cat and a little hole for the kitten! The humanities—such as reading the Greek classics—do not always make a man *humane*, that is, liberal, tolerant, gentle, and candid, as regards the opinions and status of other men.

I think the fault does not lie in any one of these or in any other of the disciplinary subjects, but in our lazy habit of using each of them as a sort of mechanical contrivance for turning up the soil and sowing the seed. But there is no reprieve on this for parents! It rests with you, even more than with the schoolmaster and his curriculum, to form those mental habits which shall give intellectual distinction to your children throughout their lives. Are you up for the great task?

You will say, perhaps, that you have already given Philip and Beatrice a great deal of training in good habits. I know that to be true, my dear—you don't need to argue your case in that matter! You have paid careful attention to their physical and also their moral habits; I am referring here, though to some *intellectual* habits which should be matters of careful training during the period of childhood. Here is a little list for you:

Attention, the power of turning the whole force of the mind upon the subject brought before it

Concentration, which differs from **Attention** in that the mind is actively engaged on some given problem rather than passively receptive

Thoroughness, the habit of dissatisfaction with a slipshod, imperfect grasp of a subject, and of mental uneasiness until a satisfying measure of knowledge is obtained

Intellectual Volition, the power, that is, of making ourselves think of a given subject at a given time (if the *child* is accustomed to take pleasure in the effort as effort, the *man* will find it easy to make himself think of what he will)

Accuracy, which is to be taught, not only through arithmetic, but through all the small statements, messages, and affairs of daily life:

Reflection, the ruminating power which is so strongly developed in children and is somehow lost with much besides of the precious cargo they bring with them into the world. There is nothing sadder than the way we allow intellectual impressions to pass over the surface of our minds, without any effort to retain or assimilate.

And I can mention only one other invaluable habit, that of **Meditation**. Now, don't laugh at that, dear Margaret, as funny as it might sound to you to think of your children deep in meditation. Meditation is also a habit to be acquired, or rather preserved, for we believe that children are born to meditate, as they are to reflect; indeed, the two are closely allied. In **reflecting** we ruminate on what we have received. In **meditating** we are not content to go over the past, we allow our minds to follow out our subject to all its issues. It has long been known that progress in the Christian life depends much upon meditation; intellectual progress, too, depends, not on mere reading or the laborious "getting up" of a subject, which we call study; but on that active surrender of all the powers of the mind to the occupation of the subject in hand, which is intended here by the word **meditation**. And of course there might be a dozen more words we could use, and thinking of some of them might keep us profitably employed for a while. But here is the question we must ask now: on what do intellectual habits sustain themselves? I think you already know the answer: the intellectual life has but one food whereby it lives and grows—the sustenance of living ideas.

It is not possible to repeat this too often or too emphatically, for perhaps we err more in this respect than any other in bringing up children. We feed them upon the white ashes out of which the last spark of the fire of original thought has long since died. We give them second-rate story books, with stale phrases, stale situations, shreds of other people's thoughts, stalest of stale sentiments. Well, we will have other opportunities to talk about what is *in* books, but let us also not forget their illustrations! We have so many opportunities to share good, meaningful art in our homes, but so many parents hang "cute" pictures in the children's rooms, and their books are illustrated on a lower level still. In regard to book illustrations, we are improving a little, but still there is room for something much better.

And in that vein, I am enclosing two little books by Miss Beatrix Potter, who now lives quite near here, at Hill Top farm in Near Sawrey. I think Philip and Beatrice (almost a namesake!) already own *The Tale of Peter Rabbit*, do they not? These two are her newest titles: *The Tale of Two Bad Mice* and *The Tale of Mrs. Tiggy-Winkle*. Please read them to the dear children with a fond embrace from their great-aunt.

(And perhaps the next post will have something in it for yourself.)

Yours affectionately…

August 4, 1904

My dear Margaret,

You have asked me about choosing more books, and I have only two things to say—first, that children have no natural appetite for twaddle, and, second, that a special literature for children is probably far less necessary than the booksellers would have us suppose. Out of any list of "the hundred best books," I believe that seventy-five would be well within the range of children of eight or nine, and not only the ones traditionally given to them. I have long been convinced that Kinglake's *Eothen* would fascinate children as much as *Robinson Crusoe*.

> *Dragoman (recovering his temper and freedom of speech).* —His Excellency, this Lord of Mudcombe, observes to your Highness, that whenever the Irish, or the French, or the Indians rebel against the English, whole armies of soldiers, and brigades of artillery, are dropped into a mighty chasm called Euston Square, and in the biting of a cartridge they arise up again in Manchester, or Dublin, or Paris, or Delhi, and utterly exterminate the enemies of England from the face of the earth.
>
> *Pasha.* —I know it—I know all—the particulars have been faithfully related to me, and my mind comprehends locomotives. The armies of the English ride upon the vapours of boiling caldrons, and their horses are flaming coals!—whirr! whirr! all by wheels!—whiz! whiz! all by steam!

[21st century editor's note: Eothen, *published in 1844 to describe a journey through the Middle East, may not suit modern tastes in various respects. Please use caution in following Miss Mason's recommendation.]*

Well, I do admit it, some of the books from the past century speak of, or to, a different world than this one, and you might choose something a little less…obscure?... for Philip and Beatrice. But let us go back to one of the true classics: *The Faerie Queene*, with its allegory and knightly adventures and sense of free moving in woodland scenery, would exactly fall in with their humour. What they want is to be brought into touch with living thought of the best, and their intellectual life feeds upon it with little meddling on our part. We do not sufficiently recognize the independent intellectual development of children which it is our business to initiate and direct, but not to control or dominate.

I know a little girl of nine who pined every day because the poems of Tennyson which she loved best were not to be found in the volumes of the larger works, which were all the house she was visiting at afforded—do you remember that? You literally missed your favourite poems as a child would miss a meal; and why not? The intellectual appetite is just as actual and just as pressing as bodily hunger; more so, alas, in some cases. And given a bountiful repast of ideas, the process of natural selection soon begins. Tennyson, with his "Our elm tree's ruddy-hearted blossom-flake is fluttering down," "Ruby-budded lime," and "Black as ash-buds in the front of March," has done more to make field botanists than any science class or examination.

Have you read the chapter about children's reading in Harriet Martineau's *Household Education?* I will guess not, since it is almost as old now as *Eothen*. Here, I have scribbled out a short passage for you:

> ...the number of ravenous readers among children is so large, and among adults so small in comparison, that I am disposed to consider it a general fact that when the faculties, naturally developed, reach a certain point of forwardness, it is the time for laying in a store of facts and impressions from books which are needed for ulterior purposes.
>
> The parents' main business during this process is to look to the quality of the books read:—I mean merely to see that the child has the freest access to those of the best quality. Nor do I mean only to such as the parent may think good for a child of such and such an age. The child's own mind is a truer judge in this case than the parents' suppositions. Let but noble books be on the shelf,—the classics of our language,—and the child will get nothing but good.

Ideas of nature, of life, love, duty, heroism–all of these!–children find and choose for themselves from the authors they read, who do more for their education than any deliberate teaching; just for this reason, that these vital ideas are self-selected and self-appropriated. As there is no religious conversion for the child who has always been brought up in the conscious presence of God, so parents who have always satisfied the intellectual craving of their children must needs forego the delight of watching a literary awakening. (But that is not such a bad thing!)

Let me conclude with a wise sentence of Coleridge's concerning the method of Plato, which should be always present to the minds of persons engaged in the training of children:—

> He desired not to assist in storing the passive mind with the various sorts of knowledge most in request, as if the human soul were a mere repository or banqueting room, but to place it in such relations of circumstance as should gradually excite its vegetating and germinating powers to produce new fruits of thought, new conceptions and imaginations and ideas.

Yrs affectionately…

P.S. I had promised to send you something for your own enjoyment, but I have had to wait on acquiring what I wanted.

Poetic Interlude #3

from *Morte D'Arthur*

by Alfred, Lord Tennyson

The old order changeth, yielding place to new,
And God fulfils Himself in many ways,
Lest one good custom should corrupt the world.
Comfort thyself: what comfort is in me?
I have lived my life, and that which I have done
May He within Himself make pure! but thou,
If thou shouldst never see my face again,
Pray for my soul. More things are wrought by prayer
Than this world dreams of. Wherefore, let thy voice
Rise like a fountain for me night and day.
For what are men better than sheep or goats
That nourish a blind life within the brain,
If, knowing God, they lift not hands of prayer
Both for themselves and those who call them friend?
For so the whole round earth is every way
Bound by gold chains about the feet of God.
But now farewell.

Study 28: Aspects of Moral Training

August 16, 1904

My dear Margaret,

You were asking about the principle of authority in the home *[Study 1]*. Perhaps parents, great as they are and should be in the eyes of their children, should always keep well to the front the fact that their authority is derived. "God does not allow" us to do thus and thus should be a rarely expressed, but often present, thought to parents who study the nature of the divine authority where it is most fully revealed, that is, in the Gospels. They see there that authority works by principles and not by rules, and as they themselves are the deputy authorities set over every household, it becomes them to consider the divine method of government. They should discern the signs of the times too, such as the current doctrine of the unknowable God—who, if He exists, does not exist for us, because we have no relations with Him. It is extremely important that parents should keep this tendency of the day in view, and counteract it if need be.

On the other hand, it is well that parents should understand the limitations of authority. Even the divine authority does not *compel.* It indicates the way and protects the wayfarer, and strengthens and directs self-compelling power. It permits a man to make free choice of obedience rather than compels him to obey. In the moral training of children, arbitrary action almost always produces revolt. Parents believe that they are doing well to *rule* their households, without considering the pattern, the principles, and the limitations of parental authority. (And we adults, so far as the nursery and schoolroom go, are we not fatally docile ourselves in yielding obedience to anyone who will take the trouble to tell *us* we had better do this or that?)

It is in their early years at home that children should be taught to realize that duty can exist only as that which we *owe* to God; that the law of God is exceeding broad and encompasses us as the air we breathe, only more so, for it reaches to our secret thoughts; and this is not a hardship but a delight. That mothers should love their little children and make them happy all day long—this is part of the law of God: that children are glad when they are good, and sad when they are naughty—this, too, is the law of God: that, if Beatrice drops her spoon and it falls to the ground, that is a law of God too, of a different kind. Mother or teacher cannot give children a better inheritance than the constant sense of being ruled and encompassed by law, and that *law* is another name for the Will of God.

Yours affectionately…

August 24, 1904

My dear Margaret,

Thank you for the loan of Adler's *The Moral Instruction of Children*. I must, however, take exception to what he writes on page 12: "It is the business of the moral instructor in the school to deliver to his pupils the subject-matter of morality, but not to deal with the sanctions of it." Here we have a contention at least two thousand years old. Protagoras preached that "Man is the measure of all things"; "Just as each thing appears to each man, so it is to him"; meaning that all truth is relative. The tendency is to think that a man can only act according to his "lights," and, therefore, that it is right for him to do that which is right in his own eyes; in other words, that every man is his own final authority in questions of right and wrong.

No doubt every child is born with a conscience, that is, with a sense that he ought to choose the right and refuse wrong; but he is not born with the power to discern good and evil. An educated conscience is a far rarer possession than we imagine; we are all startled now and then by the laxities of right-minded neighbours in matters the right and wrong of which is patent to ourselves; but probably our own moral eccentricities are equally startling to our friends. The blame rests on our faulty moral education, which has hardly made us aware of fallacious thought and insincere speech; we believe that Latin and Greek must be taught, but that morals come by *nature*. A certain rough-and-ready morality, varying with our conditions, does come by heredity and environment; but that most delicate and beautiful of human possessions, an educated conscience, comes only by teaching with authority and adorning by example.

But it is curious how educated people are still at sea as regards the moral status of children. Some time ago I was present at an interesting discussion, among the members of an educational society, on the subject of children's lies. It was interesting to notice that the meeting, consisting of able, educated people, divided itself into those who held that children were born *true* and those who held that they were born *false*; it did not occur to anybody to recall his own childhood, or even to reflect on his own condition at the present moment. The question lay between children being born *moral* and born *immoral*. Nobody reflected that every human being comes into the world with infinite possibilities for good; and, alas! infinite possibilities for evil; possibly with evil hereditary tendencies which may be rectified by education, or even with good tendencies which his bringing-up may (sadly) nullify.

Well, anyway, may I suggest an antidote to such teachings as Adler's? It is already close at hand to you, and will cost you nothing. But I think I will leave you to mull that over until my next letter.

Yours affectionately…

August 27, 1904

My dear Margaret,

No, I was not suggesting *The Tale of Two Bad Mice*, no matter how much little Beatrice has taken to it, and though we might draw a redemptive *motif* from its ending.

No, for this we need go no further than the Ten Commandments, and our Lord's exposition of the moral law, to find corrective teaching for the spasmodic, impulsive moral efforts which tend to make up our notion of what the children call "being good"; and nowhere shall we find a more lucid and practical commentary on the moral law than is set forth in the Church Catechism. It was the practice of a venerable Father of the Church, Bishop Ken, to recite the "duty towards God" and the "duty towards my neighbour" every day. It is a practice worth imitating, for children of any communion! *[Study 11]*

But, second to this, do you remember my citing of poetry as awakening children's awareness of nature, as a sort of "second nature?" Well, the poets also give us admirable help in moral teaching; as, for example, Wordsworth's *Ode to Duty*, which by the title sounds quite odious, but let us hear from it anyway:

> Stern lawgiver! yet thou dost wear
> The Godhead's most benignant grace;
> Nor know we anything so fair
> As is the smile upon thy face;
> Flowers laugh before thee on their beds;
> And fragrance in thy footing treads;
> Thou dost preserve the stars from wrong;
> And the most ancient heavens, through thee, are
> fresh and strong.

Or this, of Tennyson—

> Not once or twice in our fair island story
> The path of duty was the way to glory:
>
> He, that ... / Thro' the long gorge to the far light, has won
> His path upward and prevail'd,—
> Shall find the toppling crags of duty, scaled,
> Are close upon the shining tablelands
> To which our God Himself is moon and sun.

Possibly we could hardly do better than lead children to reflect on some high poetic teaching, adding love to law and devotion to duty, so that children shall know themselves, by duty as by prayer,

> Bound by gold chains about the feet of God.

In the matter of the ideas that inspire the virtuous life, we miss much by our way of taking things for granted. Consider the many things right around you! and begin with those.

Yours affectionately…

[On another sheet of paper]

I had intended to post my letter earlier, but as this examination response has just landed on my desk, I thought it quite relevant.

> Q. What have you noticed about a thrush? Tell all you know about it.
>
> F. (aged 8): Thrushes are browny birds. They eat snails, and they take the snail in their mouths and knock it against a stone to break the shell and eat the snail. I found a stone with a lot of bits of shell round it, so knew that a thrush had been there. Where we used to live a thrush used to sing every morning on the same tree. The song of the thrush is like a nightingale. We often see a lot of thrushes on the lawn before breakfast or after a shower. They have yellow beaks and their breasts are specked with lovely yellow and brown. Once we found a thrush asleep on a sponge in a bedroom and we carried it

> out and put it on a tree. Thrushes eat worms as well as snails, and on the lawn they listen with their heads on one side and go along as the worm gets under the ground, and presently, perhaps, the worm comes up and they gobble it up, or they put their beaks in and get it. Thrushes build their nests with sticks at the bottom and line them with little bits of wool they pick up, or feathers, and they like to get down very much.

September 3, 1904

My dear Margaret,

I promised to send you something for your own study, and so I have—were you expecting a book? Well, not this time. I have managed to get some small but good prints for you of certain medieval frescoes, so that you may do a mother's picture study, perhaps with the interested friends you have mentioned?

The medieval Church endeavoured to answer the Socratic inquiry: "What ought we to do and what do we mean by the words 'ought' and 'doing' or 'acting?'"; and it answered, as far as might be, by way of object-lessons, visible signs of spiritual things signified. Those things passed down speak to us so well of these things, if we had eyes to see and ears to listen!

What are these pictures? In the Arena (or Scrovegni) Chapel at Padua, we have Giotto's Faith and Infidelity, Love and Envy, Charity and Avarice, Justice and Injustice, Temperance and Gluttony, Hope and Despair, pictured forth in unmistakable characters for the reading of the unlearned and ignorant. I say "we have" deliberately, because this is indeed something that was given to the people, and that is still available for us to make our own.

And we have the same theme, treated with a difference, in Notre-Dame of Amiens, where we may study Humility and Pride, Temperance and Gluttony, Chastity and Lust, Charity and Avarice, Hope and Despair, Faith and Idolatry, Perseverance and Atheism, Love and Discord, Obedience and Rebellion, Courage and Cowardice, Patience and Anger, Gentleness and Churlishness,—in pairs of quatrefoils, an upper and a lower, each under the feet of an Apostle who was held to personify the special virtue. (But the words alone do not give one the true sense of why Ruskin called it "the Bible of Amiens," don't you agree?—and this is why I am sending the prints as well.)

A more recent attempt at this personification of virtue may be seen in St. Mary's Cathedral in Edinburgh, where Phoebe Traquair has frescoed the walls to illustrate the *Benedicite*, and where "holy and humble men of heart," for example, is illustrated by three men of our own day, of different schools of thought—Cardinal Newman is the only one I recollect.

> O ye Servants of the Lord, bless ye the Lord: praise him, and magnify him for ever.

> O ye Spirits and Souls of the Righteous, bless ye the Lord: praise him, and magnify him for ever.
>
> O ye holy and humble Men of heart, bless ye the Lord: praise him, and magnify him for ever.

But, outside of such rare later works, *we* know nothing about cardinal virtues and deadly sins. *We* have no teaching by authoritative utterance strong in the majesty of virtue. *We* work out no schemes of ethical teaching in marble; we paint no scale of virtues on our walls, and no repellent vices. Our poets speak for us, it is true; but the moral aphorisms, set like jewels though they be on the forefinger of time, are scattered here and there, and we leave it serenely to happy chance whether our children shall or shall not light upon the couple of lines which should fire them with the impulse to virtuous living.

It may be said that we neglect all additional ethical teaching because we "have" the Bible; but how far, and how, do we have or use even that? Here we have indeed the most perfect ethical system, the most inspiring and heart-enthralling, that the world has ever possessed; but it is questionable whether we attempt to set a noble child's heart beating with the thought that he is required to be perfect as his Father which is in Heaven is perfect. It is time we set ourselves seriously to this work of moral education which is to be done, most of all, by presenting the children with high ideals. The theme of the "moral law" suggests endless subjects for consideration and direct teaching: for example, lives chosen for a particular theme; Bible heroes; Greek heroes; moral object-lessons; etc.

"Lives of great men all remind us we can make our lives sublime," said Longfellow; and the study of the lives of "great" men, and of the great moments in the lives of "smaller" men, is most wonderfully inspiring to children. The Bible is, of course, a storehouse of most inspiring biographies; but it would be well if we could manage our teaching so as to bring out in each character the master-thought of all his thinking—that special virtue or form of endeavour which seemed to her the keynote of his character.

And of course, as with the teaching in physical and intellectual habits, we may make use not only of actual biographies, but also the burning words of the poets—Tennyson's *Ode on the Death of the Duke of Wellington*, for example.

> Lead out the pageant: sad and slow,
>
> As fits an universal woe,
>
> Let the long procession go,
>
> And let the sorrowing crowd about it grow,
>
> And let the mournful martial music blow;
>
> The last great Englishman is low.

In the reading of the Bible, of poetry, of the best prose, the culling of mottoes is a delightful and most stimulating occupation, especially if a motto book be kept, perhaps under headings, perhaps not. Beatrice is still probably too young, but it would not be a bad idea for Philip to make his own "year-book," with a motto for every day in the year culled from his own reading. If not this year, then perhaps beginning at his next birthday, and Great-Aunt Charlotte might send him a small notebook in which to copy those mottoes in beautiful lettering, perhaps as a Sunday occupation. It is something we could do for ourselves as well: what an incentive to a good day it would be to read in the morning, as a motto of our very own choice and selection, and not the voice of an outside mentor: "Keep ye the law; be swift in all obedience!"

But as we have spoken of the *ideas* of moral training, what of moral *habits*? One point, dear Margaret: you and George should take pains to have your own thoughts clear as to the manner of virtues you want the children to develop. Candour, fortitude, temperance, patience, meekness, courage, generosity, indeed the whole role of the virtues, would be stimulating subjects for thought and teaching, offering ample illustrations. The moral impulse having been given by means of some such inspiring idea as we have considered, the parent's or teacher's next business is to keep the idea well to the front, with tact and delicacy, and without insistence, and to afford apparently casual opportunities for moral effort on the lines of the first impulse.

Again, let us keep before the children that it is the manner of thoughts we think which matters; and, in the early days, when a child's face is an open book to his parents, the habit of sweet thoughts must be kept up, and every selfish, resentful, unamiable movement of children's minds observed in the countenance must be changed before consciousness sets in. One caution I should like to offer. A child's whole notion of religion is "being good." It is well that he should know that being good is *not* his whole duty to God, although it is so much of it; that the relationship of love and personal service, which he owes as a child to his Father, as a subject to his King, is even more than the being good which gives our Almighty Father such pleasure in His children.

Yours most affectionately…

Study 29: Aspects of Religious Education

September 15, 1904

My dear Margaret,

We have already spoken about religious education, or perhaps we should rather say that the other areas of teaching—the physical, the intellectual, the moral—always seem to lead back to the same place, and here we find ourselves stopping at last.

And of course whatever I can manage to add here will not by any means by exhaustive. My treatment has for its object indication of practical lines for religious education; and I very earnestly hope that you *will* find I have "left out things I ought to have said, or said things I ought not to have said."

Let us first consider how the principle of **authority** bears on religious teaching. The sense of duty, more or less illuminated, or more or less benighted, is always relative to a ruler with whom it rests to say "Thou shalt" or "Thou shalt not." This, I think, we have already firmly established, yes? *[Study 1]* It is brought home, to most of us who are set in authority, that we ourselves are acting under a higher, and finally, under the highest rule. A child cannot have a lasting sense of duty until he is brought into contact with a Supreme Authority, who is the source of law, and the pleasing of whom converts duty into joy. In these rather latitudinarian days, there is perhaps no part of religious teaching more important than to train children in the sense of the immediate presence and continual going forth of the supreme Authority. "Thou art about my path and about my bed and spiest out all my ways," as Psalm 139 has it in our Morning Prayer, should be a thought, not of fear, but of very great comfort to every child.

This constant recognition of authority excites the twofold response of *docility* and of *reverence*. It is said that the children of our day are marked by willfulness and a certain flippancy and want of reverence. If this is so, and insofar as it *is* so, it is because children are brought up without the consciousness of their *relation* to God, whom we are taught to call "Our Father." This divine name reminds us that authority is lodged in the Author of our being, and is tender, pitiful, preventive, strong to care for and wise to govern; as we see it feebly shown forth even in the best of human fathers. Yes, I said in the *best*, and I do not mean it to slight dear George, but we need to understand this as a comparison with the best that our human, limited efforts can give.

Now, something else important: there are questions in the air, in any newspaper or magazine you will pick up these days; in the Universities; even in our churches, about the authenticity of the Scriptures and what not, so that we are all more or less at the mercy of words. Many words, long words, that question the verbal accuracy of passages of the Scriptures, and that therefore give us a dim idea that the divine Authority itself is in question. We cannot fully ignore the words; but, at the same time, the Parents' Union has recognized the need to strengthen the hands of parents by comforting them with the sense of the higher Power behind theirs, and always supporting them in the exercise of the deputed powers they hold as heads of families.

There is another notion in the air which tells against the recognition of authority, and that is, the greatly increased respect for individual personality and for the right of each individual to develop on the lines of his own character. Oh, you will say, but what about the principle that "Children are born persons?" But it is a mistake to suppose that the exercise of authority runs counter to any individual development that is not on morally wrong lines. They must go hand-in-hand.

Now, as for the *ideas* that need to be taught in this regard: the supreme authority (and all deputed authority) works precisely as does a good and just national government, whose business it is to defend the liberties of the subject at all points, even by checking, repressing, and punishing the license which interferes with the rights of others and with the true liberty of the transgressor.

The law (that is, the utterance of authority) is "for the punishment of evil-doers, but for the praise of them that do well" (1 Peter 2:14); and the association of harshness, punishment, force, arbitrary dealings, with the idea of authority, human and divine, is an example of the confusion of thought to which most of our errors in conduct are traceable. It is not *authority* which punishes: the penalties which follow us through life, of which those the family are a faint foretaste, are the inevitable consequences of broken *law*, whether moral or physical, and from which authority, strong and benign, exists to save us by prevention, and, if needs be, by lesser and corrective penalties.

In regard to your mothers' group, it seems to me that reading and teaching for parents on the following subjects might help to focus thought on a subject of vital importance:

our relation to the supreme authority, not a relation of choice, but as inevitable as the family relationships into which we are born

the duty of loyalty and the shame of infidelity

the duty of reverence

the duty of docility to indications of the divine will

Scriptural revelations of God as the ruler of men, as saying to Abraham, "Go, and he goeth"; to Cyrus, "Do this, and he doeth it"

revelations which history affords of God as the ruler of nations, and as the benign ruler of men who prospers the ways of His servants

how the sense of the divine authority may be imparted in the home

and how reverence for holy things may be taught.

But how may we do that last thing? Well, if direct teaching is still somewhat out of reach, we may at least begin by laying down of lines of *habit* in the religious life, most particularly how far this power can be employed in the religious development of a child. Let us consider the subject as it bears upon habits of thought and of attitude, of life and of speech; though indeed all these are one, for every act and attitude is begotten of a thought, however unaware we be of thinking.

It is said of the wicked that "God is not in all their thoughts" (Psalm 28:5). Of the child it should be said that God is in *all* his thoughts; happy-making, joyous thoughts, restful and dutiful thoughts, thoughts of loving and giving and serving, the wealth of beautiful thoughts with which every child's heart overflows.

I must close off now, but know that my thoughts and prayers are also with you right now, especially with the soon-coming happy event.

Yours most affectionately…

September 21, 1904

My dear Margaret,

You are concerned that Philip seems a little morbid and precocious when he asks questions and has imaginings about things divine, and so you do your best to divert him. Might I suggest that diversion is not, perhaps, the best tactic in this area? What he needs is to be guided into true, happy thinking; every day should bring him "new thoughts of God, new hopes of heaven," as Keble's hymn says. Philip understands things divine better than we do, because his ideas have not been shaped yet to a conventional standard; and thoughts of God are to him an escape into the infinite from the worrying limitations, the perception of the prison bars which are among the bitter pangs of childhood. To keep a child in this habit of the thought of God—so that to lose it, for even a little while, is like coming home after an absence and finding his mother out—is a very delicate part of a parent's work.

It is most important to establish the habit of reverent attitudes—something that is a little apt to be overlooked in these days. We are, before all things, sincere, and are afraid, in teaching and raising children, to insist upon "mere forms," feeling it best to leave the child to the natural expression of his own emotions. Here, perhaps again, we are wrong, as it is just as true to say that the form gives birth to the feeling as that the feeling should give birth to the form. Children should be taught to take time, to be reverent at grace before meals, at family prayers, at their own prayers, and in church, when they are old enough to attend.

In my own young days, many children stood daily by their mother's knee, in reverent attitude, to recite the Apostles' Creed; and the recollection of the reverence expressed in that early act remains with one through a lifetime. It is a mistake to suppose that the forms of reverence need be tiresome to them. They love little ceremonies, and to be taught to kneel nicely while saying their short prayers would help them to a feeling of reverence in after-life. The habit of regularity in children's devotions is very important. The chair, or the bedside, or the little prayer-table, or, best of all, the mother's knee, plays no small part in framing the soul to a habit of devotion. In this connection it is worthwhile to remark that the evening prayers of children and of school girls and boys should not be left until the children are tired and drop asleep over their evening exercises. After tea is a very good set time for prayers when it can be managed.

The habit of hearing, and later, of reading the Bible, is one to establish at an early age. We are met with a difficulty—that the Bible is, in fact, a library containing passages and, indeed, whole books which are not for the edification of children; and many parents fall back upon little collections of texts for morning and evening use. But I doubt the wisdom of this plan. We may believe that the narrative teaching of the Scriptures is far more helpful to children, anyway, than the stimulating moral and spiritual texts picked out for them in little devotional books. We might, instead, find (or have printed) small single books of the Bible. A child such as Philip who is old enough to take pleasure in reading for himself would greatly enjoy reading through the Gospel of St. Mark, bit by bit, for example, in a nice little book, as part of his morning's devotions. (A small warning, though: while pressing the importance of habits of prayer and devotional reading, it should be remembered that children are little formalists by nature, and that they should not be encouraged in long readings or long prayers with a notion of any merit in such exercises.)

In connection with children's behaviour in church (which you have mentioned to be a problem with little Beatrice), the sentiment and forms of reverence cannot be expected if they are taken to church too young, or to too long services or are expected to maintain their attention throughout. If Beatrice must be taken to long services, she should be allowed the resource of a Sunday picture-book, and told that the hymns and the "Our Father," for example, are the parts of the service for her. If there are special worship times designed for families, this need not be as much of a problem, but as this is not always possible, we must just do our best.

Perhaps we do not attach enough importance to the habit of praise in our children's devotion. Praise and thanksgiving come freely from the young heart; gladness is natural and holy, and music is a delight. The singing of hymns at home and of the hymns and canticles in church should be a special delight; and the habit of soft and reverent singing, of offering our very best in praise, should be carefully formed.

Children should be trained in the habits of attention and real devotion during short services or parts of services. The habit of finding their places in the prayer-book and following the service is interesting and aids attention, but perhaps it would be well to tell children, of even Philip's age, that during the litany, for example, they might occupy themselves by saying over silently hymns that they know. Hymns with a story are perhaps the best for little children, like this one you will remember:

A little ship was on the sea,
It was a pretty sight;
It sailed along so pleasantly,
And all was calm and bright.

When lo! a storm began to rise,
The wind grew loud and strong;
It blew the clouds across the skies,
It blew the waves along...

He to the storm says, Peace, be still!
The raging billows cease;
The mighty winds obey His will,
And all are hushed to peace.

Oh, well we know it was the Lord,
Our Savior and our friend;
Whose care of those who trust His word
Will never, never end.

But all this question of hymn-writing for children has been much argued, since the days of Isaac Watts and Charles Wesley, and no doubt your own children will fasten on certain hymns that catch their imaginations and offer "new thoughts of God."

And finally, the habit of Sunday-keeping. Sunday stories, Sunday hymns, Sunday walks, Sunday talks, Sunday painting, Sunday knitting even, Sunday card-games, should all be special, peculiar to the day,—quiet, glad, serene. The people who clamour for a Sunday that shall be as other days little know how healing to the jaded brain is the change of thought and occupation the seventh day brings with it. There is hardly a more precious inheritance than that of the traditional English Sunday, stripped of its austerities, we hope, but keeping its character of quiet gladness and communion with Nature as well as with God.

But I cannot pursue the subject of *habits* further here. Trusting that all is well with you and yours, and that the next news we have here will be of the new arrival.

Yours most affectionately...

October 4, 1904

My dear Margaret,

Happiest welcome to babies Mildred Marie and Frank Edward! What a lovely double surprise for this great-aunt; I do not remember there being twins in our family before. I am enclosing a copy of Robert Bird's *Jesus, the Carpenter of Nazareth*, inscribed to the babies but really for all the children. (I chose that book on the recommendation of one of our *Parents' Review* writers, Mrs. Hatchell, and I am enclosing a copy of a very comprehensive article she recently submitted—do read it, when you have the time (!). A sampling:

> "Play" says [the German writer Johann Paul Friedrich Richter, also known as] Jean Paul, "is the first poetry of the child, because 'play' is its first statement of its first deeds." We also say, paradoxical as it sounds, that the first work of the child is Play...How many mothers have watched the first play of the little baby of a few months old, lying on his back, kicking his little legs, and throwing his arms in the air, combining play and exercise, and seeming the living embodiment of the poet's words that it is "a joy to be alive"; and we know how, as the months go on into years, this is but the earliest stage of that play which is the agency that gives him health; for "play" is an absolute necessity to his physical life...
>
> Do we mothers sufficiently realise the importance of our children's play, in the unconscious training and developing of certain moral qualities and powers, far more than they can be by any mere words of ours on the subject; what potent factors their games can be in teaching lessons of self-control, self-reliance, unselfishness, patience, courage and energy?
>
> Froebel says, "The first mental development of the child goes on in its play, and this play needs consequently to be as much systematised as the instruction given at a later stage."

In relation to your earlier question about Sunday occupations, she also makes a few suggestions:

> I would suggest special books only to be given out on Sundays, and not kept in the same shelf with the other books read during the week, if possible, so as to have special associations for that day. In

> fact, I often do not allow the book to be gone on with during the week, when it is wanted, but say, "Wait until next Sunday..."
>
> I think Miss Soulsby has some very practical and helpful words on this point of Sunday reading which we may apply to our children as well as to ourselves. She says, "Practically, if we do not read good books on Sunday, we do not read them at all. It is not so much that a novel is wrong on Sunday, as that better things leave no time for it... It is not a negative rule, which should keep us right, but the 'expulsive power of a new affection' at which we should aim."

Mrs. Hatchell ends with these lines:

> Let us remember, that in our children's "play" as well as in their "books," are many opportunities afforded to us of training habits which will form an important part in their lives hereafter, and let us not miss our opportunities for want of what Pestalozzi calls "a thinking love" on our part.

Still, there is a little danger, in these days of much educational effort, and even those genuine opportunities for training in habits, that children's play should be crowded out, or should be prescribed for and arranged until there is no more freedom of choice about play than that about work; and even in their *work*, we are too apt to interfere with children. We all know the delight with which any scope for personal initiative is hailed, the pleasure children take in doing anything which they may do their own way; anything, in fact, which allows room for skill of hand, play of fancy, or development of thought. With our present theories of education it seems that we cannot give much scope for personal initiative, and it is only now and then a child gets the chance to produce himself in his work. But let us use such opportunities as come in our way.

Much love from the aunt-to-all...

P.S. Will you be planning to buy one of those large perambulators so that the babies can get enough fresh air?

October 12, 1904

My dear Margaret,

Well, as to our talk on religious education for the children, the most important part of our subject remains to be considered—the inspiring *ideas* we propose to give children in the things of the divine life. This is a matter we are a little apt to leave to chance; but when we consider the vitalizing power of an idea, and how a single great idea changes the current of a life (as does the birth of twins!), it becomes us to consider very carefully what *ideas* of the things of God we may most fitly offer children, and how these may be most invitingly presented.

It is a very sad fact that many children get their first ideas of God in the nursery, and that these are of a "Being" on the watch for their transgressions and always ready to chastise. It is hard to estimate the alienation which these first ideas of the divine Father set in the hearts of His little children. Another danger is, lest the things of the divine life should be made too familiar and hackneyed, that the name of our blessed Lord should be used without reverence; and that children should get the notion that the Lord God exists for *their* uses, and not they for *His* service.

Perhaps the first vitalizing idea to give children is that of the tender fatherhood of God; that they live and move and have their being within the divine embrace. Let children grow up in this joyful assurance, and, in the days to come, infidelity to this closest of all relationships will be as shameful a thing in their eyes as it was in the eyes of the Christian Church during the age of faith.

Second, the idea of Christ their King is fitted to touch springs of conduct and to rouse the enthusiasm of loyalty in children, who have it in them, as we all know, to bestow heroic devotion on that which they find heroic. Perhaps we do not make enough of this principle of hero-worship in human nature in our teaching of religion. We are inclined to make our religious aims subjective rather than objective; to look upon Christianity as a scheme of salvation designed and carried out for our benefit; whereas the very essence of Christianity is passionate devotion to an altogether adorable Person. But, recognizing this, there is still a danger in these days of adopting a rose-water treatment of children. Few grown up people, alas! have so keen and vivid a sense of sin as a little transgressor say of six or seven. Many a naughty, passionate, or sulky and hardened little offender is so, simply because he does not know, with any personal knowledge, that there is a Saviour of the world, who has for him instant forgiveness and waiting love. But here again, the thoughts of a child should be turned *outwards* to Jesus, our Saviour, and not *inward* to his own thoughts and feelings.

One more thought is all that I have space to touch upon. Most Christian parents teach their children to recognize the indwelling of the Holy Ghost, the Comforter; they expand the ideas expressed in—

> Enable with perpetual light
> The dulness of our blinded sight.

Do you know that old hymn of John Cosin's? It is a good hymn for thoughtful Christians, but (as in Verses 3 and 4) especially for parents who, while wiping the "soiled faces," desire their children to learn the "endless song."

But it would be well if we could hinder in our children's minds the rise of a wall of separation between things sacred and things so-called secular, by making them feel that all "sound learning," as well as all "religious instruction," falls within the office of God, the Holy Spirit, the supreme educator of humankind.

And may He bless you, George, and all your dear little ones.

Ever affectionately, etc…

Study 30: Three Years Later

October 1, 1907

My dear Margaret,

You well know the Parents' Union motto, "Education is an atmosphere, a discipline, a life," especially in the diagrammatic form in which it appears on the covers of our Library books. I am told that we, as a society, are destined to live by our motto! A notable educationalist writes to me, in connection with public education: "There is more need than ever for such a view of education as that embodied in the memorable words which are the motto of the *Parents' Review*."

Well, an inspiring motto must always be a power, but to live *upon* the good repute of our motto, and to live *up* to it and *in* it, are two different things; and I am afraid the Parents' Union has much and continual thinking, and strenuous living, to face, if it proposes to stand before the world as interpreting and illustrating these "memorable words." But we are not a faint-hearted body; we *mean*, and mean intensely; and to those who purpose the best, and endeavour after the best, the best arrives.

But, in regard to that motto (and in other things), we sometimes err, I think, in taking a part for the whole, and a part of a part for the whole of that part. Of the three clauses, that which declares that "education is an atmosphere" currently pleases us most, perhaps, because it is the most inviting to the *laissez aller,* unrestrained principle of human nature. By the way, we lose something by substituting *environment* for *atmosphere.* The latter word is symbolic, it is true, but a symbol means more to us all than the name of the thing signified. We think of fresh air, pure, bracing, tonic,—of the definite act of breathing which must be fully accomplished; and we are incited to do more, and mean more, in the matter of our children's surroundings if we regard the whole as an *atmosphere*, than if we accept the more literal term *environment.* (Are you getting outside enough these days with the children? I hope it will be easier now that the twins are better able to clamber about on their own.)

But, suppose that "education is an atmosphere" brings a fresh and vigorous thought to our minds; suppose that it means to us, for our children, sunshine and green fields, pleasant rooms and good pictures, schools where learning is taken in by the gentle act of *inspiration*, followed by the *expiration* of all that which is not wanted, where charming teachers compose the children by a half-mesmeric effluence which inclines them to do as others do, be as others are,—suppose that all this is included in our notion of "education is an atmosphere," may we not sit at our ease and believe that all is well, and that the whole of education has been accomplished?

No; because though we cannot live *without* air, neither can we live *upon* air, and children brought up upon "environment" soon begin to show signs of inanition. This notion, that education is included in *environment*, or, at the best, in *atmosphere*, has held the ground for a generation or two, and it seems to me that it has left its mark upon our public and our private lives. We are more ready to be done unto than to do; we do not care for the labour of ordering our own lives in this direction or in that; they must be conducted for us; a press of engagements must compel us into what next, and what next after. We crave for spectacular entertainment, whether in the way of pageants in the streets, or spectacles on the boards. Even Shakespeare has come to be so much the occasion for gorgeous spectacles that what the poet says is of little moment compared with the show a play affords. There is nothing intentionally vicious in all this; it is simply our effort to escape from the *ennui* that results from a one-sided view of education: that education is an atmosphere only.

But, to go back further: an equally consuming *ennui* set in at the end of the eighteenth century, and that also was the result of a partial view of education. "Education is a life" was the (unconscious) formula then; and a feverish chase after *ideas* was the outcome. It is pathetic to read how Madame de Staël and her coterie, or that "blue-stocking" coterie which met at the Hôtel Rambouillet, for example, went little to bed, because they could not sleep; and spent long nights in making character sketches of each other, enigmas, anagrams, and other futilities of the intellect, and met again (some of them) at early breakfast to compose and sing little airs, upon little themes. We may be as much inclined to yawn in each other's faces as they were, but, anyway, if we sin as they did by excess in one direction, there is less wear and tear in a succession of shows than in their restless pursuit of inviting notions. (Byron wrote of Madame de Staël that she was a woman "with her pen behind her ears and her mouth full of ink.")

Still, that earlier century has its lessons for ours. They erred, as we do, because they did not understand the science of the proportion of things. We are inclined to say, "education *is* environment"; they would say, "education *is* ideas." The truth includes both of these, *plus* a third definition introducing another aspect of education. This third conceivable view, "education is a discipline," has always had its votaries, and has them still. That the discipline of the habits of the good life, both intellectual and moral, forms a good third of education, we all believe. The excess occurs when we imagine that certain qualities of character and conduct run out, a prepared product like carded wool or sausage, from this or that educational machine, mathematics or classics, science or athletics; that is, when the notion of the development of the so-called *faculties* takes the place of the more physiologically true notion of the formation of intellectual *habits. [Study 6]*

The difference does not seem to be great; but two streams that rise within a foot of one another may water different countries and fall into different seas, and a broad divergence in practice often arises from what appears to be a small difference in conception, in matters educational. The father of Plutarch had him learn his Homer so that he might get heroic ideas of life. Had the boy been "put through" Homer as a classical grind, as a machine for the development of faculty, a pedant would have come out, someone who was ostentatious about his great knowledge of the small details of his subject, and not a man of the world in touch with life at many points, capable of bringing men and affairs to the touchstone of a sane and generous mind.

It seems to me that this notion of the discipline which should develop "faculty" has tended to produce rather one-sided men, with the limitations which belong to abnormal development. An artist told me the other day that a painter must think pictures, paint pictures, nothing but pictures. But when art was great, men were not mere artists. The Flemish painter Quentin Matsys, we are told, began as a blacksmith, and then turned to painting pictures (supposedly because his wife thought painting to be a more "romantic" profession!). Michael Angelo wrote sonnets, designed buildings, painted pictures; marble was by no means his only vehicle of expression. Leonardo da Vinci wrote treatises, planned canals, played instruments of music, did a hundred things, and all exquisitely. But then, the idea of the development of *faculty*, and the consequent discipline, had not occurred to these great men, or their guardians. As I trust that you will equally and kindly ignore it in the raising of your children,

Yours affectionately…

October 8, 1907

My dear Margaret,

So, having safe-guarded ourselves from the notion that education has only one face, we can now go on to consider how "education is a life," without the risk of thinking that we are viewing more than one side of the subject. It has been said that "man doth not live by bread alone, but by every word that proceedeth out of the mouth of God" (Matt. 4:4); and the importance of the occasion on which the words were spoken has caused us to confine their meaning to what we call the life of the soul; but, indeed, they include a great educational principle which was better understood by the medieval Church than by ourselves.

Do you still have the prints I once sent you of the various frescoes? (I do hope you will be able to view them someday for yourself as well. Perhaps George might consider taking time from his work so that the two of you could take that long-delayed trip to Italy? But I digress.) Have another careful look at the Spanish Chapel fresco *[Study 10]*. At the highest point of the picture we see the Holy Ghost descending in the likeness of a dove; immediately below, in the upper chamber are the disciples who first received His inspiration; below, again, is the crowd of all nationalities who are brought indirectly under the influence of that first outpouring; and in the foreground are two or three dogs, showing that the animals were not excluded from benefiting by the new grace.

In the lower compartment of the great design are angelic figures of the cardinal virtues, which we all trace more or less to divine inspiration, floating above the seated figures of apostles and prophets, of whom we know that they "spake as they were moved by the Holy Ghost." So far, this medieval scheme of philosophy reveals no new thought to persons instructed in the elements of Christian truth. But below the prophets and apostles are a series of pictured niches, those to the right being occupied by the captain figures, the ideal representations, of the seven Liberal Arts, figures of singular grace and beauty, representing such familiar matters as grammar, rhetoric, logic, music, astronomy, geometry, and arithmetic, all of them under the same divine outpouring which illuminated the disciples in the upper chamber.

Now here is a very large truth: our nature craves after unity. You can see it in the play of your little children, and you know it to be true in your own self. The travail of thought which is going on to-day, and has gone on as long as we have any record of men's thoughts, has been with a view to establishing some principle for the unification of life. And here, in this painting, we have the scheme of a magnificent unity. Just as we tried to separate out "education is an atmosphere" and "education is a life," we are apt to think that piety is one thing, that our intellectual and artistic yearnings are quite another matter, and that our moral virtues are pretty much matters of inheritance and environment, and have not much to do with our conscious religion. Hence, there come discords into our lives, discords especially trying to young and ardent souls who want to be good and religious, but who cannot escape from the overpowering drawings of art and intellect and mere physical enjoyment; they have been taught to consider that these things are, for the most part, alien to the religious life, and that they must choose one or the other; they do choose, and the choice does not always fall upon those things which, in our unscriptural and unphilosophical narrowness, we call the things of God.

And think of this: Michael Angelo writes that "in order to represent the adored image of our Lord, it is not enough that a master should be great and able. I maintain that he must also be a man of good morals and conduct, if possible a saint, in order that the Holy Ghost may give him inspiration." In truth, a nation or a human being becomes great upon one diet only, the diet of great ideas communicated to those already prepared to receive them by a higher Power than Nature herself.

Yours affectionately…

October 23, 1907

My dear Margaret,

Our Chapel reading this morning included St. Paul's words that "A little leaven leaveneth the whole lump (Galatians 5:9)." It made me think that our Parents' Union holds amongst us such a little leaven, and that you parents have the same opportunity as you raise your children. Let us all then set ourselves to labour with purpose and passion to restore to the world, enriched by the additions of later knowledge, that great scheme of unity of life which produced great men and great work in the past.

(Ah, the later knowledge? I thought you would not miss that.)

Nor need we fear that in endeavouring after some such doctrine of ideas as may help us in the work of education, we are running counter to science. And now you see where this letter is going.. Many of us feel, and, I think, rightly, that the teaching of science is *the* new teaching which is being vouchsafed to humankind in our age. Some of us are triumphant, and believe that the elements of moral and religious struggle are about to be eliminated from life, which shall run henceforth, whether happy or disastrous, on the easy plane of the inevitable. Others look in vain for a middle way, a place of reconciliation; while others of us, again, take refuge in repudiating "evolution" and all its works, and nailing our colours to "religion," interpreted on our own narrow lines. Whichever of these lines we take, we probably err through want of *faith*.

Let us first of all settle it with ourselves that science and religion cannot, to the believer in God, by any possibility be antagonistic. Having assured ourselves of this (yes, it is possible!), we shall probably go on to perceive that the evolution of science is in fact a process of revelation, being brought about in every case, so far as I am aware, by the process which Coleridge has so justly described; that is,

> where the *ideas* of nature (presented to chosen minds by a Higher Power than nature herself) suddenly unfold, as it were, in prophetic succession, systematic views destined to produce the most important revolutions in the state of man!

I know we are not much in sympathy with Huxley *[Study 9]*, but it is interesting that he describes Biology "as helping to give right ideas in this world, which is, after all," he goes on to say, "absolutely governed by ideas, and very often by the wildest and most hypothetical ideas." Again, he writes, "those who refuse to go beyond the fact rarely get as far as the fact; and anyone who has studied the history of science knows that almost every great step therein has been made by the 'anticipation of nature,' that is, by the invention of hypotheses." Things have to unfold, don't they? But, as he says, we also have to get ourselves "as far as the fact." One cannot help thinking that scientists would find the unifying principle they are in search of in the fine saying of Coleridge's; so would they stand revealed to themselves as the mouthpieces, not merely of *the truth*, for which they are so ready to combat and suffer, but also as the chosen and prepared servants of Him who is the Truth.

Your loving aunt…

October 28, 1907

My dear Margaret,

So, you ask what I meant by "Evolution as the Master-Thought of the Age?"

For three thousand years thinkers have been occupied with attempts to explain the world by means of a single principle, which should also furnish an explanation of reason and the human soul. Heraclitus and his age thought they had laid hold of the informing idea in the phrase, "The true Being is an eternal Becoming"; the "universal flux of things" explained all. Democritus and his followers "solved" the riddle of the universe with the saying that "nothing exists except atoms moving in vacancy." Many times since, with each epoch-making discovery, has science cried "Eureka!" over the one principle which should explain all things—and eliminate Personality.

But some little knowledge of history and philosophy will give us pause. We shall see that each great discovery, each luminous idea of nature that the world has received hitherto, is like a bend in a tortuous lake which appears final until your boat approaches it, and then–behold an opening into further and still further reaches beyond! And the knowledge of God will give us something more than the wider outlook which comes of a knowledge of history–the knowledge that there *is* what Wordsworth calls the "stream of tendency," a stream of immeasurable force in shaping character and events; but there is also Personality, a power able to turn the stream of tendency to its uses, if also liable to be carried away in its current.

I believe that the keyword for the interpretation of life, both animal and vegetable, has been presented to our generation, and we cannot overrate the enormous repose and satisfaction to the human mind contained in the idea of *evolution*. Are you properly horrified? Well, my dear, the idea planted its feet a good forty years or more ago, so I do not believe we can view its influence as only a *fad*. If I appear to dwell on a subject which at first sight appears to have little to do with the bringing up of children, it is because I think that our attitude towards the great idea, great lesson, set for our own age to grasp, is a vital part of a parent's preparation. If parents take no heed of the great thoughts which move their age, they cannot expect to retain influence over the minds of their children. If they fear and distrust the revelations of science, they introduce an element of distrust and discord into their children's lives.

But if, with the mere neophyte of science, they rush to the conclusion that the last revelation is final, that it accounts for all that is in man, and, to say the least, makes God unnecessary and unknowable, or negligible, they may lower the level of their children's living to that struggle for existence–without aspiration, consecration, and sacrifice–of which we hear so much. If, lastly, parents recognize every great idea of nature as a new page in the progressive revelation made by God to men already prepared to receive such an idea; if they realise that the new idea, however comprehensive, is *not* final nor all-inclusive, nor to be set in opposition with that personal knowledge of God which is the greatest knowledge, why, then, their children will grow up in that attitude of reverence for science, reverence for God, and openness of mind, which befits us for whom life is a probation and a continual education.

So much for the nutriment of ideas laid on the table of the world during *this* particular course of its history. And what next? We may have poetry, or art, or philosophy; we cannot tell; but two things are incumbent upon us—to keep ourselves and our children in touch with the great thoughts by which the world has been educated in the past, and to keep ourselves and them in the right attitude towards the great ideas of the present.

Your always-affectionate aunt,

Charlotte M. Mason.

Notes for a New Era

What ideas move this generation?

In January 2021, Rowan Williams wrote this in *The New Statesman:*

> The *New Statesman*'s weekly back-page Q&A always ends with the question: "Are we all doomed?" There is a simple sense in which the answer is "yes". There is nothing we love or value that we shall not eventually have to give up, there is no life-project that does not have an expiry date.
>
> The more interesting question is whether we can imagine not just giving up but "giving over"—finding the energy to hand on what we love and value, to enhance lives that will outlast ours. And for this to happen we have to have space and skills to explore what those things are, to love what "we must leave ere long", as Shakespeare's sonnet puts it. It is time for us to think again about all our educational institutions and practices in that light.

Charlotte Mason identified three key ideas, or cultural narratives, or "schoolmasters of the world," from the early twentieth century *[Study 6]*: the sacredness of the person, the evolution of the individual, and the solidarity of the (human) race.

What are those things that you love and value? Do they seem to match the ideas of your culture, or contradict them? And where do they come from?

> In a world of proliferating choice (consumer choice, that is), we are less prone [than we used to be] to feel we are deprived of an identity we value. In fact, it is likely that someone is trying very hard to understand what we feel is authentic so that it can be packaged somehow and sold to us in the form of a rebellious T-shirt or self-help book. (Plumb, 2009, pp. 5-14)

Even if our personal values conflict with the ideas of this age (as Miss Mason wrote to Margaret), we must still be aware of what is blowing through the world, in order to speak to it. Is there some facet of current thought that *does* line up with "education is the science of relations?" Or "education is an atmosphere, a discipline, and a life?" With the principle that "children are born persons?"

(Self)-Teaching Through Play

In the *Parents' Review* article quoted, Mrs. Hatchell writes,

> Do we mothers sufficiently realise the importance of our children's play, in the unconscious training and developing of certain moral qualities and powers, far more than they can be by any mere words of ours on the subject; what potent factors their games can be in

> teaching lessons of self-control, self-reliance, unselfishness, patience, courage and energy?

Miss Mason has said elsewhere *[Study 11]* that children's free play must not be meddled with by their elders, and Mrs. Hatchell agrees:

> I can bear this out in my own experience, for on several occasions when I have unwittingly interrupted my little daughter's play of this description, by letting my amused feelings get the better of me, and thus making her conscious of my presence; I notice she does not pick up the thread again till I have gone away, or pretend to be absorbed in a book, and then the imaginary conversations begin again, revealing many curious workings and reproductions of the childish mind.

However, it seems that what Mrs. Hatchell is recommending is not so much a conscious effort on the part of the parent to manipulate or "use" a child's play as the training ground for a checklist of moral lessons, as simply a recognition that the activity of play *does* teach these things, and that if we recognize its importance, we will do our best to provide "means and opportunity" for it.

The Third Corner

> We are inclined to say, "education *is* environment"; they would say, "education *is* ideas." The truth includes both of these, *plus* a third definition introducing another aspect of education. This third conceivable view, "education is a discipline," has always had its votaries, and has them still.

Miss Mason believed that choosing one's favourite of the first two led to imbalance; but that adding the third corner–so to speak–would complete the educational triangle. Why did she think that "education is a discipline" was so necessary? What limit must we put on it?

Epilogue: In Which Miss Mason Has the Last Word

"Many unlikely things happen in life," said Frau Sesemann with a pleased smile. "Two things coming together may produce a happy result, as for instance, a fresh zeal for learning and a new method of teaching, and neither does any harm. We can but rejoice that the child has made such a good start and hope for her future progress." (*Heidi*, by Johanna Spyri)

That normal children have a natural desire for, and a right of admission to, all knowledge, appears to me to be covered by the phrase, 'Education is the science of relations.' (Charlotte Mason, Preface to *School Education*, November 1904)

In considering the training of children under the convenient divisions of *physical*, *intellectual*, *moral*, and *religious*, I have not thought it necessary to give counsels upon matters of common knowledge and general acceptance, but have dwelt upon aspects of training under each heading which are rather likely to be overlooked. Under the phrase "Education is a life," for example, I have tried to show how necessary it is to sustain the intellectual life upon ideas, and, as a corollary, that a school-book should be a medium for ideas and not merely a receptacle for facts.

It is our temptation to make too personal a matter of education, to lose sight of the fact that education is a world business, that the lessons of the ages have been duly set, and that each age is concerned, not only with its own particular page, but with every preceding page. For who feels that he has mastered a book if he is familiar with only the last page of it? This brings me to a point I am anxious to bring forward. We do not sufficiently realize the need for unity of principle in education. We have no Captain Idea which shall marshal for us the fighting host of educational ideas which throng the air; so, in default of a guiding principle, a leading idea, we feel ourselves at liberty to pick and choose. This man thinks he is free to make science the sum of his son's education; the other chooses the classics; a third prefers a mechanical, and a fourth, a commercial programme; a fifth makes bodily health his cult, and chooses a school which makes the care of health a special feature of its programme (not that we must allow health to be neglected, but that, given good general conditions, the less obvious attention their health receives the better for the boys and girls); and everyone feels himself at liberty to do that which is right in his own eyes with regard to the education of his children.

Now, here is the danger that besets us in education. We as teachers seize upon "child study" as applied to mind; upon terrible agglutinations which we call "apperception masses" *[Study 7]*; upon intellectual futilities in a hundred directions, each of which will, we hope, give us the key to education. We may perceive the futility of such notions by applying the test of progress. Are they the way *to* anything, and, if so, to what? It is exciting to become a pioneer; but, for the children's sake, it may be well to constrain ourselves to follow those roads *only* by which we know that persons have arrived; or those newer roads which offer evident and assured means of progress towards a desired end. Self-will is not permitted to the educationalist; and he may not take up fads. Let it be our negative purpose to discourage in every way we can the educational faddist, that is, the person who accepts a one-sided notion in place of a universal idea as his educational guide.

But let us try, however imperfectly, to make education a science of relationships—in other words, try in one subject or another to let the children work upon living ideas. In this field small efforts are honoured with great rewards, and we perceive that the education we are giving exceeds all that we intended or imagined.

Charlotte Mason's Principles of Education; or, This Book in Three Pages

(Principles as listed in *Philosophy of Education*)

> "No sooner doth the truth...come into the soul's sight, but the soul knows her to be her first and old acquaintance."
>
> "The consequence of truth is great; therefore the judgment of it must not be negligent." *(both quotations by Benjamin Whichcote)*

1. Children are born *persons*.

2. They are not born either good or bad, but with possibilities for good and evil.

3. The principles of authority on the one hand and obedience on the other, are natural, necessary and fundamental; but—

4. These principles are limited by the respect due to the personality of children, which must not be encroached upon, whether by fear or love, suggestion or influence, or undue play upon anyone natural desire.

5. Therefore we are limited to three educational instruments—the atmosphere of environment, the discipline of habit, and the presentation of living ideas.

6. When we say that "*education is an atmosphere,*" we do not mean that a child should be isolated in what may be called a 'child-environment' especially adapted and prepared, but that we should take into account the educational value of his natural home atmosphere, both as regards persons and things, and should let him live freely among his proper conditions. It stultifies a child to bring down his world to the child's level.

7. By "*education is a discipline,*" we mean the discipline of habits, formed definitely and thoughtfully, whether habits of mind or body. Physiologists tell us of the adaptation of brain structures to habitual lines of thought, i.e., to our habits.

8. In saying that "*education is a life,*" the need of intellectual and moral as well as of physical sustenance is implied. The mind feeds on ideas, and therefore children should have a generous curriculum.

9. We hold that the child's mind is no mere sac to hold ideas; but is rather, if the figure may be allowed, a spiritual organism, with an appetite for all knowledge. This is its proper diet, with which it is prepared to deal; and which it can digest and assimilate as the body does foodstuffs.

10. Such a doctrine as e.g. the Herbartian, that the mind is a receptacle, lays the stress of education (the preparation of knowledge in enticing morsels duly ordered) upon the teacher. Children taught on this principle are in danger of receiving much teaching with little knowledge; and the teacher's axiom is , 'what a child learns matters less than how he learns it.'

11. But we, believing that the normal child has powers of mind which fit him to deal with all knowledge proper to him, give him a full and generous curriculum; taking care only that all knowledge offered him is vital, that is, that facts are not presented without their informing ideas. Out of this conception comes our principle that,—

12. *"Education is the Science of Relations"*; that is, that a child has natural relations with a vast number of things and thoughts: so we train him upon physical exercises, nature lore, handicrafts, science and art, and upon many living books, for we know that our business is not to teach him all about anything, but to help him to make valid as many as may be of—

> "Those first-born affinities
> "That fit our new existence to existing things."

13. In devising a SYLLABUS for a normal child, of whatever social class, three points must be considered:

(a) He requires *much* knowledge, for the mind needs sufficient food as much as does the body.

(b) The knowledge should be various, for sameness in mental diet does not create appetite (*i.e.,* curiosity)

(c) Knowledge should be communicated in well-chosen language, because his attention responds naturally to what is conveyed in literary form.

14. As knowledge is not assimilated until it is reproduced, children should 'tell back' after a single reading or hearing: or should write on some part of what they have read.

15. A *single reading* is insisted on, because children have naturally great power of attention; but this force is dissipated by the re-reading of passages, and also, by questioning, summarising. and the like.

Acting upon these and some other points in the behaviour of mind, we find that the *educability of children is enormously greater than has hitherto been supposed*, and is but little dependent on such circumstances as heredity and environment.

Nor is the accuracy of this statement limited to clever children or to children of the educated classes: thousands of children in Elementary Schools respond freely to this method, which is based on the *behaviour of mind.*

16. There are two guides to moral and intellectual self-management to offer to children, which we may call 'the way of the will' and 'the way of the reason.'

17. *The way of the will:* Children should be taught, (a) to distinguish between 'I want' and 'I will.' (b) That the way to will effectively is to turn our thoughts from that which we desire but do not will. (c) That the best way to turn our thoughts is to think of or do some quite different thing, entertaining or interesting. (d) That after a little rest in this way, the will returns to its work with new vigour. (This adjunct of the will is familiar to us as *diversion*, whose office it is to ease us for a time from will effort, that we may 'will' again with added power. The use of *suggestion* as an aid to the will is to be *deprecated*, as tending to stultify and stereotype character, It would seem that spontaneity is a condition of development, and that human nature needs the discipline of failure as well as of success.)

18. *The way of reason:* We teach children, too, not to 'lean (too confidently) to their own understanding'; because the function of reason is to give logical demonstration (a) of mathematical truth, (b) of an initial idea, accepted by the will. In the former case, reason is, practically, an infallible guide, but in the latter, it is not always a safe one; for, whether that idea be right or wrong, reason will confirm it by irrefragable proofs.

19. Therefore, children should be taught, as they become mature enough to understand such teaching, that the chief responsibility which rests on them *as persons* is the acceptance or rejection of ideas. To help them in this choice we give them principles of conduct, and a wide range of the knowledge fitted to them. These principles should save children from some of the loose thinking and heedless action which cause most of us to live at a lower level than we need.

20. We allow no separation to grow up between the intellectual and 'spiritual' life of children, but teach them that the Divine Spirit has constant access to their spirits, and is their Continual Helper in all the interests, duties and joys of life.

Appendix A: English Grammar Lesson

Subject: English Grammar.

Group: Language. Class II. Average age: 10.

Time: 20 minutes.

OBJECTS.

1. To increase the children's power of reasoning and attention.
2. To increase their knowledge of English Grammar.
3. To introduce a new part of speech—preposition.

LESSON.

Step 1. Draw from the children the names of the two kinds of verbs and the difference between them, by putting up sentences on the board. Thus in the sentence 'Father slept,' 'slept,' as they know, is intransitive; therefore he could not 'slept' anything, as 'slept' cannot have an object.

Step 2. Put on the board the sentence 'Mary went,' and ask the children to try and make it more complete by adding an object. 'Mary went school' would not make sense, but 'Mary went to school' would. Ask for other phrases saying where Mary went, as, for a walk, into the town, with mother, on her bicycle, by train, etc.

Step 3. Tell the children that these little words, on, in, by, for, with, etc., belong to a class of words which are very much used with intransitive verbs; they have not much meaning when used alone, yet in a sentence they cannot stand without an object. You cannot say 'Mary went in,' without saying what she went in.

Step 4. Introduce the word 'preposition,' giving its derivation. Because these little words always take objects after them, and because their place is before the object, they are called prepositions, 'pre' being the Latin word for 'before,' and 'position' another word for 'place.'

Step 5. Write on the board the definition:— 'A pre-position always has an object after it.'

Step 6. Let the children work through the following exercises:

(1) Put three objects after each of the following prepositions:—in, on, over, by, with, and from.

(2) Put three prepositions and their objects after the following:—Mary plays, Mother sits, John runs.

(3) Supply three prepositions in each of the following sentences:—The book is __ the table. The chair is __ the door. I stood __ the window.

(4) Supply three subjects and verbs to each of the following prepositions and objects: __ in the garden, __ on the floor, __ by the fire.

(5) Make three sentences about each of the following, each sentence to contain an intransitive verb, a preposition and its object:—The white pony, My little brother, That pretty flower.

Appendix B: German Grammar Lesson

Subject: German Grammar.
Group: Languages. Class III. Average age: 13.
Time: 30 minutes.

OBJECTS.

1. To show the pupil that although the German construction of sentences may seem very much complicated, yet with the help of a few simple rules it can be made much clearer.
2. To draw these rules from the pupil by means of examples.
3. To teach two or three of these elementary rules.
4. To strengthen the relationship with the foreign language.

LESSON.

Step 1. Begin by finding out what the pupils know of compound sentences in English, i.e. that they consist of two or more clauses depending on each other, etc., and let them give one or two examples. Connect this lesson with a former one on the arrangement of words in German sentences by letting the pupils put one or two compound clauses on the board in German, and then giving the rule they illustrate.

Rule. Dependent clauses take the verb at the end of the clause.

These sentences the pupils can probably give themselves.
Step 2. Get the old rule that the past participle comes at the end of the sentence, with a few examples, one or two of which the pupils may write upon the board to compare with those illustrating the new rule.
Let the pupils put sentences on the board illustrating the new rule.

Rule. In dependent clauses the auxiliary follows the past participle.

Sentences.— 'Ich kehre zurück, wenn sie angekommen ist.'
'Das Kind, welches verloren war, ist gefunden.'

Let the pupils translate these literally into English, and with the German clauses already on the board and the translation let them find the rule. Let them translate a few sentences into German to show that they thoroughly understand the rule.

Step 3. Treat the next rule almost in the same way, but have each sentence put on the board twice in different order, and find the rule by comparing these.

Rule. If the subordinate clause comes first the principal clause takes its verb at the beginning.

Sentences:—
'Sie gab den Armen viel, weil sie gut war!'
'Weil sie gut war, gab sie den Armen viel.'
'Er ging immer fort, obwohl er müde war.'
'Obwohl er müde war, ging er immer fort.'

Step 4. Recapitulate.

Appendix C: Two History Lessons

Subject: The Godwins.
Group: History. Class III. Average age: 13.

OBJECTS.

1. To recapitulate and enlarge on the period of history taken during the term (A.D. 871-1066).
2. To increase interest in it by giving as much as possible the history of one of the prominent families of the period.
3. To exemplify patriotism in the character of the Godwins.

LESSON.

Step 1. Recapitulate what the girls know of the period briefly by questioning about the Saxon and the Danish kings and leading men, making a chart on the blackboard.
Step 2. Begin with the reign of Canute. Enlarge upon their present knowledge as to his character and deeds whilst king of England, and let a girl read the account of his pilgrimage to Rome (Freeman's *History*, p. 242).
Step 3. Give an account of the early history of Earl Godwin…Put on the blackboard the names of the three divisions of England, with their earls or rulers.
Step 4. …Canute's treatment of the people of Worcester and the conduct of Godwin and the other earls on that occasion (p. 250).
Step 5. Edward the Confessor. Ask them questions about his early life and education, and how these affected his character and ideas. Was he a suitable man for a king? Not powerful enough to rule—Godwin became his supporter and adviser. Marriage of Godwin's daughter, Edith, to the king. Godwin's eloquence and influence over the people. (Read from Knight's *History*, p. 162.)
Step 6. Godwin's patriotism is put to the test.
Step 7. Godwin's return…Harold a worthy successor.
Show from a map the divisions of England at the death of the 'Confessor.' Read from Lord Lytton's *Harold* (p. 63).

Subject: History.
Class IV. Age: 16.

THE STATE OF FRANCE IN 1789.

OBJECTS.

1. To establish relations with the past.
2. To show how closely literature and history are linked together and how the one influences the other.

3. To try to give yet a clearer idea of the social and political state of France before the Revolution than the girls have now, and to draw from them the causes which brought about the Revolution (1789).

LESSON.

Step 1. Begin by noticing the state of France generally. Feudalism was still in existence, without its usefulness and with most of its abuses, and it led to the great division of Classes …
Step 2. Speak of the state of France in the country, showing what was the relation of the peasant to his lord…
Step 3. Notice the state of France in the towns, showing how impossible it was for a poor man to set up in a trade…
Step 4. The state of the Church…
Step 5. Show that these evils might have been remedied gradually (as in England) had there been a representative assembly regularly called, or any true justice…
Step 6. Draw from the students the reason why the Revolution broke out in France rather than in any other Continental country…
Step 7. Draw from the students why the Revolution broke out just in 1789…Get from them something of Louis' character.
Step 8. A short recapitulation of the principal points.

Appendix D: The Study of Words

Q. Distinguish between arrogant and presumptuous, interference and interposition, genuine and authentic, hate and detest, loathe and abhor, education and instruction, apprehend and comprehend, using each word in a sentence.

E. (aged 15):— "A man who is 'arrogant' is a man who has right to what he wants, but who is harsh and exacting in taking it. A 'presumptuous' man is a man who expects more than is due and takes it. 'Judge Jeffries was an arrogant old man.' 'Charles II. was a presumptuous king, he thought he could have absolute power.'

'Interference,' is not minding your own business, and meddling with other people's when we are not wanted. 'Interposition' is more the 'doing good by interfering' as protecting a little boy from a bully. 'But for the interference of James all would have gone well.' 'Thanks to the interposition of Mary a quarrel was averted.'

"Genuine' means real, true, what it seems to be as— 'a real genuine ruby.' 'Authentic,' in speaking of a book, means really written by the author to which it is ascribed. 'Dickens' Oliver Twist is certainly authentic!'

"You would 'hate' a man who killed your father. 'Charles II. hated Cromwell.' You would 'detest' a man who had not done you any personal injury, but who *(sic)* you knew to be a murderer. 'Yeo *detested* the Spaniards.'

"You would 'loathe' a poisonous snake or a hypocrite. 'David Copperfield *loathed* Uriah Heep!' You would abhor a man inferior to you in intellect or principles, as a great king would 'abhor' a cringing coward, leave him behind, go on without him, refuse to listen to him. 'Napoleon *abhorred* the traitor.'

"'Education' is the lessons you receive as a matter of course, as French, writing, grammar. 'Instruction' is this, but more also, it includes moral teaching, the teaching of honesty, and the teaching of gentleness. 'Henry had a good education.' 'No well-instructed Britain (sic) is a coward.'"

"'Apprehend' is to see, or hear, and notice. 'Comprehend' is to understand, without seeing or hearing perhaps. 'Phillip *apprehended* that danger was near, but he did not *comprehend* it.'"

Bibliography

Part One: Books by and about Charlotte Mason

Cholmondeley, E. (2021). *The Story of Charlotte Mason, 1842-1923.* Bristol, England: Lutterworth Press.

Mason, C. M. (1906/1989). *Formation of character.* Reprint, with foreword by by John Thorley. Wheaton, IL: Tyndale House.

Mason, C. M. (1886/1989). *Home education.* Reprint, with foreword by John Thorley. Wheaton, IL: Tyndale House.

Mason, C. M. (1905/1989). *Ourselves.* Reprint, with foreword by by John Thorley. Wheaton, IL: Tyndale House.

Mason, C. M. (1896). *Parents and children.* Reprint, with foreword by by John Thorley. Wheaton, IL: Tyndale House.

Mason, C. M. (1925/1989). *A philosophy of education.* Reprint, with foreword by John Thorley. Wheaton, IL: Tyndale House.

Mason, C. M. (1904/1989). *School education.* Reprint, with foreword by John Thorley. Wheaton, IL: Tyndale House.

Part Two: The Edwardian Bookcase

Adams, J. (1897). *The Herbartian psychology applied to education.* London, England: D.C. Heath & Co.

Adler, F. (1900). *The moral instruction of children.* London, England: Edward Arnold.

Arnold-Forster, H.O (1897). *A history of England from the landing of Julius Caesar to the present day.* London, England: Cassell & Co. Ltd.

Beecher, H.W. (1862). *Eyes and ears.* Boston, MA: Ticknor and Fields.

Bird, R. (1892). *Jesus, the carpenter of Nazareth.* London, England: Kegan Paul, Trench, Trubner & Co., Ltd.

Boswell, J. (1904). *Boswell's life of Johnson in two volumes.* Edinburgh, Glasgow, New York, and Toronto: Henry Frowde.

Bremer, F. & Howitt, M. (trans.) (1883). *The neighbours: A story of every-day life.* London, England: George Bell & Sons.

Browning, R. (1904) *Pocket volume of selections from the poetical works of Robert Browning.* London, England: Smith, Elder.

Buckley, A. (1899). *The fairy-land of science.* London, England: Edward Stanford.

Buckley, A. (1901). *Plant life in field and garden.* London, England: Cassell & Co. Ltd.

Bullen, F.T. (1903). *The cruise of the "Cachalot": Round the world after sperm whales.* London, England: Smith, Elder & Co.

Byron, Lord (1904). *The poetical works of Lord Byron.* London, England: Henry Frowde.

Carlyle, T. (1887). *Heroes, hero-worship and the heroic in history.* New York, NY: John B. Alden Publishing.

Chaucer, G., Spenser, E., & Purves, D.L. (ed.) (1889). *The Canterbury tales and faerie queene, with other poems of Chaucer and Spenser.* Edinburgh, Scotland: W. P. Nimmo, Hay, & Mitchell.

Child, L.M. (1836). *The American frugal housewife: Dedicated to those who are not ashamed of economy.* Boston, MA: American Stationers' Company.

Church of England (1885).*The book of common prayer, and administration of the sacraments, and other rites and ceremonies of the church, etc.* Published by Henry Frowde; Oxford University, England.

Coleridge, S.T. (187-). *A dissertation on the science of method, or, the laws and regulative principles of education.* London, England: Griffin.

Coleridge, S.T. (1851). *General introduction to the encyclopaedia metropolitana; or, a preliminary treatise method.* London, England: —.

Coleridge, S.T. (1904) *Aids to reflection and the confessions of an inquiring spirit.* London, England: George Bell & Sons.

Collingwood, W.G. (1903). *Ruskin relics.* London, England: Isbister & Company Limited.

Creighton, L. (1904). *A first history of France*. London, England: Longmans, Green & Co.

De Quincey, T., & Masson, D. (ed.) (1897). *Collected writings of Thomas De Quincey*. London, England: A.& C. Black.

Freeman, E.A. (1901). *Old English history*. London, England: Macmillan and Co.

Holden, E.S. (1903). *The sciences: A reading book for children*. Boston, MA & London, England: Ginn & Co.

Huxley, T.H. (1900). *Physiography: An introduction to the study of nature*. London, England: Macmillan and Co.

Ingelow, J.(1900). *Poems*. London, England: George Routledge.

James, W. (1905). *Psychology*. New York, NY: Henry Holt.

Kidd, B. (1894). *Social evolution*. London, England: Macmillan.

Kinglake, A.W. (1904). *Eothen*. Edinburgh, Scotland: William Blackwood and Sons.

Kingsley, C. (1902). *Madam how and lady why or first lessons in earth lore for children*. London, England: Macmillan.

Kipling, R. (1899). *Poems and ballads*. New York, NY: H.M. Caldwell.

Knight, C. (1881) *Popular history of England.* New York, NY: J.W. Lovell.

Lamb, C., & Ainger, A. (ed.) (1899). *Essays of Elia, in Life and works of Charles Lamb Vol. 1*. London, England: Macmillan.

Latham, H. (1904). *Pastor pastorum, or the schooling of the apostles by our Lord.* Cambridge, England: D. Bell and Co.

Lawrence of the Resurrection, Brother, & Smith, H.W. (1899). *The practice of the presence of God: Being conversations and letters of Nicholas Herman of Lorraine (translated from the French).* London, England: James Nisbet & Co.

Locke, J. (1854). *The works of John Locke: Philosophical works, with a preliminary essay and notes by J.A. St. John.* London, England: Henry G. Bohn.

Lockyer, J.N (1881). *Elementary lessons in astronomy*. London, England: ??.

Lytton, E.B., Baron (1893). *Harold.* Boston, MA: Little, Brown.

Luther, M. & Evangelical Lutheran Church in the United States, General Synod (1893). *Luther's small catechism etc.* Philadelphia, PA: Lutheran Publication Society.

Magnus, P. (1903). Handwork and headwork in elementary schools: A forecast. In *Educational Aims and Efforts, 1880-1910* (1910). London, England: Longmans, Green & Co.

Martineau, H. (1849). *Household education.* Philadelphia, PA: Lea & Blanchard.

Miall, L.C. (1904). *House, garden and field: a collection of short nature studies.* London, England : Edward Arnold. (And other works)

Milton, J., & Masson, D.(1907). *Poetical Works of John Milton.* London, England: Macmillan & Co.

Plutarch & North, T. (trans.) (1894/5). *Lives of the noble Grecians and Romans.* London, England: Dent.

Rein, W. (1895). *Outlines of pedagogics. Translated by C.C. and Ida J. Van Liew, with additional notes by the former.* Syracuse, NY: C.W. Bardeen.

Rogers, S., & Sargent, E. (ed.) (1854). *The complete poetical works of Samuel Rogers, with a biographical sketch and notes.* Boston, MA: Phillips, Simpson & Co.

Ruskin, J. (19--?). *Works.* New York, NY: T.Y. Crowell.

Schofield, A.T. (1891). *Physiology for Schools.* London, England: Cassell & Co..

Scott, W. (1897). *Waverley, or, 'tis sixty years since.* London, England: Adam & Charles Black.

Shakespeare, W., & Clarke, C. & M.C. (eds.) (1886?). *The plays of William Shakespeare.* London, England: Cassell & Co.

Sonnenschein, A. (1876). *The A B C of arithmetic (Teacher's book).* London, England: Whittaker and Company.

Spencer, H. (1886). *Education: Intellectual, moral and physical.* Boston, MA: Willard Small.

Spencer, H. (1886). *Essays: Moral, political and aesthetic.* New York, NY: D. Appleton

Sterne, L. (1903). *A sentimental journey*. London, England: Cassell.

Tennyson, A. (Lord) (1909). *Works of Alfred Lord Tennyson*. London, England: Macmillan & Co.

Trench, R.C., & Palmer, A.S. (1905). *On the study of words*. London, England: Routledge & Sons.

Trevelyan, G.O. (1905). *Life and letters of Lord Macaulay*. London, England: Longmans, Green and Co.

Wordsworth, W. (1904). *The prelude or growth of a poet's mind*. London: J.M. Dent.

Wordsworth, W., & Hutchinson, T. (ed.) (1904). *The poetical works of William Wordsworth*. London, Edinburgh, Glasgow, New York, Toronto: Henry Frowde.

Part Three: Useful Additions

Enright, E.(1969). *The Saturdays*. New York, NY: Henry Holt.

Fisher, D. C. (1917). *Understood Betsy*. New York, NY: Grosset & Dunlap.

Pride, M. (1994). *Schoolproof*. Wheaton, IL: Crossway Books.

Taylor, S. (1996). *All-of-a-kind family*. New York, NY: Random House Children's Publishing.

Part Four: Periodicals and Other Media

Breckenridge, D. (2021). Biographical sketch of William Wordsworth. In Breckenridge, D. et al. (Series Ed.), *AmblesideOnline poetry anthology*. Privately published.

Hatchell, Mrs. (1906). Our children's play: their toys and books. *The parents' review, 17*, No. 5, 366-??. (May be read on the AmblesideOnline website.)

Jacobs, A. (2022, February 2). Myths and counter-myths [Web log message]. Retrieved from https://blog.ayjay.org/myths-and-counter-myths/

Jacobs, A. (2022, February 8). On attentional norms: The inevitability of Zooming while distracted. [Web log message] Retrieved from https://hedgehogreview.com/web-features/thr/posts/on-attentional-norms

Plumb, D. (Winter 2009). Critical adult education in Canada in the time of CASAE. *New Directions For Adult & Continuing Education,* No. 124, 5-14.

Williams, R. (2021, January 27). Notes on a crisis: With Covid and the climate crisis, we are failing the next generation. *The New Statesman.* Retrieved from https://www.newstatesman.com/politics/2021/01/notes-crisis-covid-and-climate-crisis-we-are-failing-next-generation

Biography

Anne E. White (www.annewrites.ca) is an Advisory member of AmblesideOnline. She is the author of *Ideas Freely Sown: The Matter and Method of Charlotte Mason*; *Honest, Simple Souls: An Advent Meditation with Charlotte Mason*; *Minds More Awake: The Vision of Charlotte Mason*; and the books of the Plutarch Project series.

Made in United States
Orlando, FL
04 November 2026

90203417R00127